INSTANT POT COOKBOOK 2022

TASTY AND ON A BUDGET RECIPES

GRETA BROWN

Table of Contents

Crunchy Mushrooms.......10
Wrapped Shrimp.......12
Lentils Spread.......14
Paprika Cranberry Dip.......15
Citrus Onion Spread.......16
Zucchini and Squash Dip.......17
Garlic Cauliflower Dip.......19
Broccoli Spread.......21
Cumin Cheese Spread.......22
Leeks and Bell Pepper Spread.......24
Chicken, Spinach and Avocado Salad.......26
Pesto Barley Bowls.......27
Balsamic Olives Salsa.......28
Cheese Dip with Peppers.......29
Juicy Chicken Drumettes.......30
Creamy Cauliflower Bites.......31
Yummy Baby Carrots.......33
Cheesy Keto Dip.......34
Simple Brussels Sprouts.......36
Quick Spinach Dip.......37

Asparagus with Mayo Dip 38
Keto Greens Dip 39
Cocktail Sausages Asian-Style 41
Stuffed Mushrooms with Cheese 43
Family Meatballs 45
Fresh Keto Meatballs 47
Preparation Time: 20 minutes 49
Delicious Cauliflower Tots 51
Keto Broccoli Balls 53
Cheesy Taco Dip 54
Meatballs with Cheese 56
Spanish Fat Bombs 58
Yummy Cocktail Wieners 60
Fresh Brussels Sprouts with Aioli Sauce 62
Cheesy Bacon Bites 63
Juicy Meatballs 65
Perfect Chicken Wings 67
2-Ingredients Chicken Wings 69
Sticky Chicken Wings 71
Simple Boiled Peanuts 73
Southern Boiled Peanuts 75
Hard Boiled Eggs 77
Steamed Artichokes 78
Zingy Boiled Peanuts 80

Unique Party Food 82
Decadent Liver Pâté 84
Exotic Mushroom Pâté 86
Garden Fresh Salsa 88
Party Meatballs 90
Cheese Loaded Burgers 92
Mini Sausage Bites 94
Refreshing Curd 96
The Best Jam Ever 97
Divine Pears 98
Berry Marmalade 99
Orange Delight 100
Simple Squash Pie 101
Winter Pudding 103
Banana Dessert 105
Apple Cake 107
Special Vanilla Dessert 109
Tasty and Amazing Pear Dessert 110
Cranberries Jam 111
Lemon Jam 112
Special Dessert 113
Spicy Cannellini Bean Salad with Dates 113
Savory Vegetarian Sandwiches 116
Eat-me" Squash and Sweet Potato Creamy Soup 118

Green Pea Medley 119
Spicy Veggie and Adzuki Bean Soup 121
Italian-Style Asparagus Salad 123
Pumpkin Porridge with Dried Cherries 125
Easy Vegan Risotto 127
Refreshing Bean Salad 129
Root Vegetable and Noodle Soup 131
Quinoa Pilaf with Cremini Mushrooms 133
Butternut Squash and Barley Bowl 135
Colorful Veggie and Coconut Soup 137
Broccoli and Carrots with Peanut Sauce 139
Delicious Old-Fashioned Chili 141
Traditional Russian Borscht 143
Winter Curry Cabbage 145
The Easiest Hummus Ever 147
Green Beans with Shiitake Mushrooms 149
Lentil Chipotle Curry 151
Chorizo Pinto Beans 153
White Beans Curry 155
Chicken and Brown Rice 156
Veg Rice 158
Mung Bean Curry 160
Mexican Rice 162
Pea & Corn Rice 164

Lentil Risotto 166
Cilantro Rice 167
Almond Risotto 169
Black Bean Burrito 170
Red Bean Curry 172
Chickpea Rice 174
Fennel Risotto 175
Black Bean Gravy 177
Mushrooms Risotto 178
Lentils Spinach Stew 179
Chorizo Red Beans 181
Coconut Risotto 183
Potato Rice 184
Bean Mustard Curry 186
White Bean Curry 188
Pea & Corn Rice 190
Shrimp & Rice Paella 192
Black Beans with Chorizo 194
Brown Chicken Rice 196
Mushroom Risotto 198
Mexican-Style Rice 200
Beef Rice 202
Cauliflower Risotto 204
Vegetable & Corn Rice 206

Yellow Potato Rice....208
Mung Bean Curry....210
Chickpea Tacos....212
Three-Bean Stew....214
Corn Lentil Stew....216

Crunchy Mushrooms

Preparation Time: 10 minutes

Servings 4

Nutritional Values per serving: 91 Calories; 6.4g Fat; 5.5g Total Carbs; 5.2g Protein; 2.8g Sugars

Ingredients

- 2 tablespoons butter, melted
- 20 ounces button mushrooms, brushed clean
- 2 cloves garlic, minced
- 1 teaspoon dried basil
- 1 teaspoon dried rosemary
- 1 teaspoon dried sage
- 1 bay leaf
- Sea salt, to taste
- 1/2 teaspoon freshly ground black pepper
- 1/2 cup water
- 1/2 cup broth, preferably homemade
- 1 tablespoon soy sauce
- 1 tablespoon fresh parsley leaves, roughly chopped

Directions

1. Press the “Sauté” button to heat up your Instant Pot. Once hot, melt the butter and sauté the mushrooms and garlic until aromatic.

2. Add seasonings, water, and broth. Add garlic, oregano, mushrooms, thyme, basil, bay leaves, veggie broth, and salt and pepper to your instant pot.
3. Secure the lid. Choose "Manual" mode and High pressure; cook for 5 minutes. Once cooking is complete, use a quick pressure release; carefully remove the lid.
4. Arrange your mushrooms on a serving platter and serve with cocktail sticks. Bon appétit!

Wrapped Shrimp

Preparation time: 5 minutes

Cooking time: 6 minutes

Servings: 4

Ingredients:

1 pound shrimp, peeled and deveined

1 cup tomato sauce

A drizzle of olive oil

8 ounces bacon slices

1 teaspoon chili powder

A pinch of salt and black pepper

Directions:

1. In a bowl, mix the shrimp with the oil, salt, pepper and chili powder and toss.
2. Set the instant pot on Sauté mode, add the shrimp and cook for 2 minutes.
3. Transfer the shrimp to a bowl, cool it down and wrap each in a bacon slice.
4. Put the tomato sauce in your instant pot, arrange wrapper shrimp inside, put the lid on and cook on High for 4 minutes.
5. Release the pressure fast for 5 minutes, arrange the shrimp on a platter and serve.

Nutritional Values per serving: Calories 162, fat 3, fiber 4, carbs 7, protein 6

Lentils Spread

Preparation time: 10 minutes

Cooking time: 20 minutes

Servings: 6

Ingredients:

- 20 ounces tomatoes, crushed
- 3 garlic cloves, minced
- 1 and ½ cups red lentils, rinsed
- A pinch of salt and black pepper
- 1 tablespoon chives, chopped
- 1 tablespoon lemon juice
- 1 and ½ cups low-sodium veggie stock

Directions:

1. In your instant pot, mix the tomatoes with the lentils, salt, pepper and the stock, put the lid on and cook on High for 20 minutes.
2. Release the pressure naturally for 10 minutes, transfer the lentils mix to a food processor, add the rest of the ingredients except the chives, pulse well, divide into small bowls, sprinkle the chives on top and serve.

Nutritional Values per serving: Calories 167, fat 4, fiber 3, carbs 8, protein 6

Paprika Cranberry Dip

Preparation time: 6 minutes

Cooking time: 15 minutes

Servings: 4

Ingredients:

- 2 and ½ teaspoons lemon zest, grated
- 1 teaspoon chili powder
- 1 teaspoon sweet paprika
- 12 ounces cranberries
- ¼ cup orange juice

Directions:

1. In your instant pot, combine all the ingredients, put the lid on and cook on High for 15 minutes.
2. Release the pressure fast for 6 minutes, blend the mix using an immersion blender, divide into bowls and serve as a dip.

Nutritional Values per serving: Calories 141, fat 2, fiber 4, carbs 5, protein 4

Citrus Onion Spread

Preparation time: 5 minutes

Cooking time: 7 minutes.

Servings: 4

Ingredients:

- 1 cup cream cheese, soft
- A pinch of salt and black pepper
- 1 tablespoon olive oil
- 6 spring onions, chopped
- Juice of 1 orange
- 1 cup water

Directions:

1. In a bowl, combine the cream cheese with spring onions and the rest of the ingredients except the water, whisk well and transfer to a ramekin.
2. Add the water in the instant pot, add the trivet inside, place the ramekin in the pot, put the lid on and cook on Low for 7 minutes.
3. Release the pressure fast for 5 minutes and serve the spread right away.

Nutritional Values per serving: Calories 120, fat 2, fiber 3, carbs 5, protein 4

Zucchini and Squash Dip

Preparation time: 5 minutes

Cooking time: 15 minutes

Servings: 4

Ingredients:

- 1 yellow onion, chopped
- 1 tablespoon olive oil
- 1 and ½ pounds zucchini, chopped
- 1 butternut squash, peeled and roughly chopped
- ½ cup veggie stock
- 1 tablespoon lemon juice
- 1 tablespoon basil, chopped
- 2 garlic cloves, minced
- 1 tablespoon mint, chopped

Directions:

1. Set your instant pot on Sauté mode, add the oil, heat it up, add the onion and garlic, stir and cook 4 minutes.
2. Add zucchinis and the rest of the ingredients except the basil and the mint, put the lid on and cook on High for 10 minutes.
3. Release the pressure fast for 5 minutes, blend the mix using an immersion blender, divide into bowls and serve with mint and basil sprinkled on top.

Nutritional Values per serving: Calories 170, fat 5, fiber 3, carbs 4, protein 6

Garlic Cauliflower Dip

Preparation time: 10 minutes

Cooking time: 15 minutes

Servings: 4

Ingredients:

- 1 yellow onion, chopped
- 1 tablespoon olive oil
- A pinch of salt and black pepper
- 1 tablespoon rosemary, chopped
- 3 garlic cloves, minced
- ½ cup chicken stock
- 1 pound cauliflower florets
- ½ cup coconut cream
- 1 tablespoons parsley, chopped

Directions:

1. Set your instant pot on Sauté mode, add the oil, heat it up, add the onion, stir and cook for 5 minutes.
2. Add the rest of the ingredients except the cream and parsley, put the lid on and cook on High for 10 minutes.
3. Release the pressure naturally for 10 minutes, add the cream, blend the mix using an immersion blender, divide into bowls, sprinkle the parsley on top and serve as a party dip.

Nutritional Values per serving: Calories 170, fat 3, fiber 2, carbs 6, protein 7

Broccoli Spread

Preparation time: 10 minutes

Cooking time: 12 minutes

Servings: 4

Ingredients:

- 2 tablespoons avocado oil
- 8 garlic cloves, minced
- ½ cup veggie stock
- 6 cups broccoli florets
- A pinch of salt and black pepper
- 3 tablespoons cream cheese, soft

Directions:

1. Set your instant pot on Sauté mode, add the oil, heat it up, add the garlic and brown for 2 minutes.
2. Add the rest of the ingredients except the cream cheese, put the lid on and cook on Low for 10 minutes.
3. Release the pressure naturally for 10 minutes, transfer the broccoli mix to a blender, add the cream cheese, pulse well, divide into bowls and serve as a party spread.

Nutritional Values per serving: Calories 178, fat 3, fiber 3, carbs 5, protein 8

Cumin Cheese Spread

Preparation time: 5 minutes

Cooking time: 8 minutes

Servings: 4

Ingredients:

- 1 teaspoon olive oil
- 1 red onion, chopped
- 2 spring onions, chopped
- 1 cup cream cheese, soft
- 2 teaspoons cumin, ground
- ¼ teaspoon red pepper flakes
- A pinch of salt and black pepper
- 1 cup water

Directions:

1. In a bowl, combine the cream cheese with spring onions and the rest of the ingredients except the water, whisk really well and put everything in a ramekin.
2. Add the water to your instant pot, add the trivet and put the ramekin inside.
3. Put the lid on, cook on Low for 8 minutes, release the pressure fast for 5 minutes and serve the spread right away.

Nutritional Values per serving: Calories 170, fat 2, fiber 3, carbs 6, protein 8

Leeks and Bell Pepper Spread

Preparation time: 10 minutes

Cooking time: 15 minutes

Servings: 6

Ingredients:

- ¼ cup veggie stock
- 1 pound red bell peppers, chopped
- 4 leeks, sliced
- A pinch of salt and black pepper
- 1 tablespoon olive oil
- 1 tablespoon lemon juice
- 2 tablespoons cream cheese
- 2 garlic cloves, minced
- 1 tablespoon cilantro, chopped

Directions:

1. In your instant pot, combine the bell peppers with the leeks and the rest of the ingredients except the cream cheese and cilantro, put the lid on and cook on High for 15 minutes.
2. Release the pressure naturally for 10 minutes, transfer the mix to a blender, add the cream cheese and pulse well.
3. Divide into bowls and serve as a spread with the cilantro sprinkled on top.

Nutritional Values per serving: Calories 180, fat 4, fiber 3, carbs 7, protein 9

Chicken, Spinach and Avocado Salad

Preparation time: 10 minutes

Cooking time: 15 minutes

Servings: 4

Ingredients:

- 1 avocado, pitted, peeled and cubed
- 2 tablespoons Greek yogurt
- 2 tablespoons mayonnaise
- 2 spring onions, chopped
- 1 and ½ cups baby spinach
- 1 cup chicken stock
- A pinch of salt and black pepper
- 1 pound chicken breast, skinless, boneless and cubed

Directions:

1. In your instant pot, combine the chicken with salt, pepper and the stock, put the lid on and cook on High for 15 minutes.
2. Release the pressure naturally for 10 minutes, drain the chicken, transfer it to a bowl, add the rest of the ingredients, toss, divide into small bowls and serve as an appetizer.

Nutritional Values per serving: Calories 224, fat 12, fiber 4, carbs 7, protein 12

Pesto Barley Bowls

Preparation time: 5 minutes

Cooking time: 20 minutes

Servings: 4

Ingredients:

- 1 cup hulled barley, rinsed
- 2 cups veggie stock
- ¾ cup basil pesto
- 1 tablespoon chives, chopped
- 1 red onion, chopped
- 1 celery stalks chopped
- A pinch of salt and black pepper

Directions:

1. In your instant pot, combine the barley with the stock, salt and pepper, toss, put the lid on and cook on High for 20 minutes.
2. Release the pressure fast for 5 minutes, stir the barley, transfer to a bowl, add the rest of the ingredients and toss well.
3. Divide into cups and serve as an appetizer.

Nutritional Values per serving: Calories 172, fat 4, fiber 4, carbs 7, protein 9

Balsamic Olives Salsa

Preparation time: 5 minutes

Cooking time: 5 minutes

Servings: 4

Ingredients:

- 1 tablespoon balsamic vinegar
- 1 tablespoon olive oil
- 1 cup cherry tomatoes, halved
- 2 green onions, chopped
- 2 cups kalamata olives, pitted and chopped
- 1 handful basil leaves, chopped
- 1 handful parsley leaves, chopped

Directions:

1. Set your instant pot on Sauté mode, add the oil, heat it up, add the tomatoes and the rest of the ingredients, toss, put the lid on and cook on High for 5 minutes.
2. Release the pressure fast for 5 minutes, divide the salsa into bowls and serve cold as an appetizer.

Nutritional Values per serving: Calories 152, fat 2, fiber 3, carbs 6, protein 7

Cheese Dip with Peppers

Preparation Time: 10 minutes

Servings 8

Nutritional Values per serving: 237 Calories; 20.6g Fat; 3.1g Total Carbs; 10.2g Protein; 1.8g Sugars

Ingredients

- 1 tablespoon butter
- 2 red bell peppers, sliced
- 1 teaspoon red Aleppo pepper flakes
- 1 cup cream cheese, room temperature
- 2 cups Colby cheese, shredded
- 1 teaspoon sumac
- 2 garlic cloves, minced
- 1 cup chicken broth
- Salt and ground black pepper, to taste

Directions

1. Press the "Sauté" button to heat up your Instant Pot. Once hot, melt the butter. Sauté the peppers until just tender.
2. Add the remaining ingredients; gently stir to combine.
3. Secure the lid. Choose "Manual" mode and High pressure; cook for 3 minutes. Once cooking is complete, use a quick pressure release; carefully remove the lid.
4. Serve with your favorite keto dippers. Bon appétit!

Juicy Chicken Drumettes

Preparation Time: 15 minutes

Servings 8

Nutritional Values per serving: 237 Calories; 20.6g Fat; 3.1g Total Carbs; 10.2g Protein; 1.8g Sugars

Ingredients

- 2 pounds chicken drumettes
- 1 stick butter
- 1 tablespoon coconut aminos
- Sea salt and ground black pepper, to taste
- 1/2 teaspoon dried dill weed
- 1/2 teaspoon dried basil
- 1 teaspoon hot sauce
- 1 tablespoon fish sauce
- 1/2 cup tomato sauce
- 1/2 cup water

Directions

1. Add all ingredients to your Instant Pot.
2. Secure the lid. Choose "Poultry" mode and High pressure; cook for 10 minutes. Once cooking is complete, use a natural pressure release; carefully remove the lid.
3. Serve at room temperature and enjoy!

Creamy Cauliflower Bites

Preparation Time: 25 minutes

Servings 8

Nutritional Values per serving: 157 Calories; 12.1g Fat; 3.6g Total Carbs; 8.9g Protein; 1.2g Sugars

Ingredients

- 1 head of cauliflower, broken into florets
- 2 tablespoons butter
- Coarse sea salt and white pepper, to taste
- 1/2 teaspoon cayenne pepper
- 1 garlic clove, minced
- 1/2 cup Parmesan cheese, grated
- 1 cup Asiago cheese, shredded
- 2 tablespoons fresh chopped chives, minced
- 2 eggs, beaten

Directions

1. Add 1 cup of water and a steamer basket to the Instant Pot. Now, add cauliflower to the steamer basket.
2. Secure the lid. Choose "Manual" mode and High pressure; cook for 3 minutes. Once cooking is complete, use a quick pressure release; carefully remove the lid.
3. Transfer the cauliflower to a food processor. Add the remaining ingredients; process until everything is well incorporated.
4. Shape the mixture into balls. Bake in the preheated oven at 400 degrees F for 18 minutes. Bon appétit!

Yummy Baby Carrots

Preparation Time: 10 minutes

Servings 8

Nutritional Values per serving: 94 Calories; 6.1g Fat; 5.9g Total Carbs; 1.4g Protein; 3.1g Sugars

Ingredients

- 28 ounces baby carrots
- 1 cup chicken broth
- 1/2 cup water
- 1/2 stick butter
- 2 tablespoons balsamic vinegar
- Coarse sea salt, to taste
- 1/2 teaspoon red pepper flakes, crushed
- 1/2 teaspoon dried dill weed

Directions

1. Simply add all of the above ingredients to your Instant Pot.
2. Secure the lid. Choose "Manual" mode and High pressure; cook for 3 minutes. Once cooking is complete, use a quick pressure release; carefully remove the lid.
3. Transfer to a nice serving bowl and serve. Enjoy!

Cheesy Keto Dip

Preparation Time: 10 minutes

Servings 10

Nutritional Values per serving: 280 Calories; 20.4g Fat; 3.7g Total Carbs; 20.6g Protein; 2.5g Sugars

Ingredients

- 10 ounces cream cheese
- 10 ounces Pepper-Jack cheese
- 1 pound tomatoes, pureed
- 10 ounces pancetta, chopped
- 1 cup green olives, pitted and halved
- 1/2 teaspoon garlic powder
- 1 teaspoon dried oregano
- 1 cup chicken broth
- 4 ounces Mozzarella cheese, thinly sliced

Directions

1. Combine cream cheese, Pepper-Jack cheese, tomatoes, pancetta, olives, garlic, powder, and oregano in your Instant Pot.
2. Secure the lid. Choose “Manual” mode and High pressure; cook for 4 minutes. Once cooking is complete, use a quick pressure release; carefully remove the lid.
3. Top with Mozzarella cheese; cover and let it sit in the residual heat. Serve warm or at room temperature. Bon appétit!

Simple Brussels Sprouts

Preparation Time: 10 minutes

Servings 4

Nutritional Values per serving: 68 Calories; 3.3g Fat; 5.8g Total Carbs; 3.5g Protein; 1.9g Sugars

Ingredients

- 1 tablespoon butter
- 1/2 cup shallots, chopped
- 3/4 pound whole Brussels sprouts
- Sea salt, to taste
- 1/4 teaspoon ground black pepper
- 1/2 cup water
- 1/2 cup chicken stock

Directions

1. Press the "Sauté" button to heat up your Instant Pot. Once hot, melt the butter and sauté the shallots until tender and translucent.
2. Add the remaining ingredients to the Instant Pot.
3. Secure the lid. Choose "Manual" mode and High pressure; cook for 4 minutes. Once cooking is complete, use a quick pressure release; carefully remove the lid.
4. Transfer Brussels sprouts to a serving platter. Serve with cocktail sticks and enjoy!

Quick Spinach Dip

Preparation Time: 5 minutes

Servings 10

Nutritional Values per serving: 43 Calories; 1.7g Fat; 3.5g Total Carbs; 4.1g Protein; 1.3g Sugars

Ingredients

- 1 pound spinach
- 4 ounces Cottage cheese, at room temperature
- 4 ounces Cheddar cheese, grated
- 1 teaspoon garlic powder
- 1/2 teaspoon shallot powder
- 1/2 teaspoon celery seeds
- 1/2 teaspoon fennel seeds
- 1/2 teaspoon cayenne pepper
- Salt and black pepper, to taste

Directions

1. Add all of the above ingredients to your Instant Pot.
2. Serve warm or at room temperature. Bon appétit!
3. Secure the lid. Choose "Manual" mode and High pressure; cook for 1 minute. Once cooking is complete, use a quick pressure release; carefully remove the lid.

Asparagus with Mayo Dip

Preparation Time: 5 minutes

Servings 6

Nutritional Values per serving: 116 Calories; 8.5g Fat; 6.9g Total Carbs; 4.5g Protein; 2.4g Sugars

Ingredients

- 1 ½ pounds asparagus spears, trimmed
- 1/2 cup sour cream
- 1/2 cup mayonnaise
- 2 tablespoons fresh chervil
- 2 tablespoons scallions, chopped
- 1 teaspoon garlic, minced
- Salt, to taste

Directions

- Add 1 cup of water and a steamer basket to you Instant Pot.
- Secure the lid. Choose "Manual" mode and High pressure; cook for 1 minute. Once cooking is complete, use a quick pressure release; carefully remove the lid.
- Then, thoroughly combine the remaining ingredients to make your dipping sauce. Serve your asparagus with the dipping sauce on the side. Bon appétit!

Keto Greens Dip

Preparation Time: 10 minutes

Servings 10

Nutritional Values per serving: 153 Calories; 10.6g Fat; 5g Total Carbs; 8.7g Protein; 3.1g Sugars

Ingredients

- 2 tablespoons butter, melted
- 20 ounces mustard greens
- 2 bell peppers, chopped
- 1 white onion, chopped
- 1 teaspoon garlic, minced
- Sea salt and ground black pepper, to taste
- 1 cup chicken stock
- 8 ounces Neufchâtel cheese, crumbled
- 1/2 teaspoon dried thyme
- 1/2 teaspoon dried dill
- 1/2 teaspoon turmeric powder
- 3/4 cup Romano cheese, preferably freshly grated

Directions

1. Add the butter, mustard greens, bell peppers, onion, and garlic to the Instant Pot.
2. Secure the lid. Choose "Manual" mode and High pressure; cook for 3 minutes. Once cooking is complete, use a quick pressure release; carefully remove the lid.
3. Then, add the remaining ingredients and press the "Sauté" button. Let it simmer until the cheese is melted; then, gently stir this mixture until everything is well incorporated.
4. Serve with your favorite low-carb dippers.

Cocktail Sausages Asian-Style

Preparation Time: 10 minutes

Servings 8

Nutritional Values per serving: 330 Calories; 24.8g Fat; 2.7g Total Carbs; 22.7g Protein; 1.2g Sugars

Ingredients

- 1 teaspoon sesame oil
- 20 mini cocktail sausages
- 1/2 cup tomato puree
- 1/2 cup chicken stock
- 1 tablespoon dark soy sauce
- 1/3 teaspoon ground black pepper
- 1/2 teaspoon paprika
- Himalayan salt, to taste
- 1/2 teaspoon mustard seeds
- 1/2 teaspoon fennel seeds
- 1/4 teaspoon fresh ginger root, peeled and grated
- 1 teaspoon garlic paste

Directions

1. Simply throw all ingredients into your Instant Pot.
2. Secure the lid. Choose "Manual" mode and High pressure; cook for 4 minutes. Once cooking is complete, use a quick pressure release; carefully remove the lid.
3. Serve with cocktail sticks and enjoy!

Stuffed Mushrooms with Cheese

Preparation Time: 10 minutes

Servings 5

Nutritional Values per serving: 151 Calories; 9.2g Fat; 6g Total Carbs; 11.9g Protein; 3.6g Sugars

Ingredients

- 1 tablespoon butter, softened
- 1 shallot, chopped
- 2 cloves garlic, minced
- 1 ½ cups Cottage cheese, at room temperature
- 1/2 cup Romano cheese, grated
- 1 red bell pepper, chopped
- 1 green bell pepper, chopped
- 1 jalapeno pepper, minced
- 1/2 teaspoon dried basil
- 1/2 teaspoon dried oregano
- 1/2 teaspoon dried rosemary
- 10 medium-sized button mushrooms, stems removed

Directions

1. Press the "Sauté" button to heat up your Instant Pot. Once hot, melt the butter and sauté the shallots until tender and translucent.
2. Stir in the garlic and cook an additional 30 seconds or until aromatic. Now, add the remaining ingredients, except for the mushroom caps, and stir to combine well.
3. Then, fill the mushroom caps with this mixture.
4. Add 1 cup of water and a steamer basket to you Instant Pot. Arrange the stuffed mushrooms in the steamer basket.
5. Secure the lid. Choose "Manual" mode and High pressure; cook for 5 minutes. Once cooking is complete, use a quick pressure release; carefully remove the lid.
6. Arrange the stuffed mushroom on a serving platter and serve. Enjoy!

Family Meatballs

Preparation Time: 15 minutes

Servings 6

Nutritional Values per serving: 384 Calories; 22.2g Fat; 6.1g Total Carbs; 38.4g Protein; 3.6g Sugars

Ingredients

- 1/2 pound ground pork
- 1 pound ground beef
- 1/2 cup Romano cheese, grated
- 1/2 cup pork rinds, crushed
- 1 egg, beaten
- Coarse sea salt and ground black pepper, to taste
- 1 teaspoon granulated garlic
- 1/2 teaspoon cayenne pepper
- 1/2 teaspoon dried basil
- 1/4 cup milk, lukewarm
- 1 ½ cups BBQ sauce

Directions

1. Thoroughly combine ground meat, cheese, pork rinds, egg, salt, black pepper, garlic, cayenne pepper, basil, and milk in the mixing bowl.
2. Then, roll the mixture into 20 meatballs.
3. Pour BBQ sauce into your Instant Pot. Now, add the meatballs and secure the lid.
4. Choose "Manual" mode and High pressure; cook for 8 minutes. Once cooking is complete, use a quick pressure release; carefully remove the lid. Bon appétit!

Fresh Keto Meatballs

Preparation Time: 15 minutes

Servings 6

Nutritional Values per serving: 280 Calories; 20.4g Fat; 3.7g Total Carbs; 20.6g Protein; 2.5g Sugars

Ingredients

- 1/2 pound ground pork
- 1/2 pound ground turkey
- 2 eggs
- 1/3 cup almond flour
- Sea salt and ground black pepper, to taste
- 2 garlic cloves, minced
- 1 cup Romano cheese, grated
- 1 teaspoon dried basil
- 1/2 teaspoon dried thyme
- 1/4 cup minced fresh mint, plus more for garnish
- 1/2 cup beef bone broth
- 1/2 cup tomatoes, puréed
- 2 tablespoons scallions

Directions

1. Thoroughly combine all ingredients, except for broth, tomatoes, and scallions in a mixing bowl.
2. Shape the mixture into 2-inch meatballs and reserve.
3. Add beef bone broth, tomatoes, and scallions to your Instant Pot. Place the meatballs in this sauce.
4. Secure the lid. Choose "Manual" mode and High pressure; cook for 8 minutes. Once cooking is complete, use a quick pressure release; carefully remove the lid. Bon appétit!
5. Parmigiano Chicken Wings

Preparation Time: 20 minutes

Servings 12

Nutritional Values per serving: 443 Calories; 30.8g Fat; 6.2g Total Carbs; 33.2g Protein; 3.5g Sugars

Ingredients

- 4 pounds chicken wings cut into sections
- 1/2 cup butter, melted
- 1 tablespoon Italian seasoning mix
- 1/2 teaspoon onion powder
- 1/2 teaspoon garlic powder
- 1 teaspoon paprika
- 1/2 teaspoon coarse sea salt
- 1/2 teaspoon ground black pepper
- 1 cup Parmigiano-Reggiano cheese, shaved
- 2 eggs, lightly whisked

Directions

1. Add chicken wings, butter, Italian seasoning mix, onion powder, garlic powder, paprika, salt, and black pepperto your Instant Pot.
2. Secure the lid. Choose "Poultry" mode and High pressure. Cook the chicken wings for 10 minutes. Once cooking is complete, use a natural pressure release; carefully remove the lid.
3. Mix Parmigiano-Reggiano cheese with eggs. Spoon this mixture over the wings.
4. Secure the lid. Choose "Manual" mode and High pressure; cook for 4 minutes longer. Once cooking is complete, use a quick pressure release; carefully remove the lid. Bon appétit!

Delicious Cauliflower Tots

Preparation Time: 25 minutes

Servings 6

Nutritional Values per serving: 132 Calories; 8.7g Fat; 4.5g Total Carbs; 9.2g Protein; 1.3g Sugars

Ingredients

- 1 head of cauliflower, broken into florets
- 2 eggs, beaten
- 1 shallot, peeled and chopped
- 1/2 cup Swiss cheese, grated
- 1/2 cup Parmesan cheese, grated
- 2 tablespoons fresh coriander, chopped
- Sea salt and ground black pepper, to taste

Directions

1. Start by adding 1 cup of water and a steamer basket to your Instant Pot.
2. Arrange the cauliflower florets in the steamer basket.
3. Secure the lid. Choose "Manual" mode and High pressure; cook for 3 minutes. Once cooking is complete, use a quick pressure release; carefully remove the lid.
4. Mash the cauliflower and add the remaining ingredients. Form the mixture into a tater-tot shape with oiled hands.
5. Place cauliflower tots on a lightly greased baking sheet. Bake in the preheated oven at 390 degrees F approximately 20 minutes; make sure to flip them halfway through the cooking time.
6. Serve at room temperature. Bon appétit!

Keto Broccoli Balls

Preparation Time: 25 minutes

Servings 8

Nutritional Values per serving: 137 Calories; 9.5g Fat; 4.8g Total Carbs; 8.9g Protein; 1.5g Sugars

Ingredients

- 1 head broccoli, broken into florets
- 1/2 cup Añejo cheese,shredded
- 1 ½ cups Cotija cheese,crumbled
- 3 ounces Ricotta cheese, cut into small chunks
- 1 teaspoon chili pepper flakes

Directions

1. Add 1 cup of water and a steamer basket to the Instant Pot.
2. Place broccoli florets in the steamer basket.
3. Secure the lid. Choose "Manual" mode and Low pressure; cook for 5 minutes. Once cooking is complete, use a quick pressure release; carefully remove the lid.
4. Add the broccoli florets along with the remaining ingredients to your food processor. Process until everything is well incorporated.
5. Shape the mixture into balls and place your balls on a parchment-lined baking sheet. Bake in the preheated oven at 390 degrees F for 15 minutes. Bon appétit!

Cheesy Taco Dip

Preparation Time: 10 minutes

Servings 12

Nutritional Values per serving: 275 Calories; 23.7g Fat; 2.6g Total Carbs; 12.4g Protein; 1.2g Sugars

Ingredients

- 2 teaspoons sesame oil
- 1/2 cup yellow onion, chopped
- 1 pound ground turkey
- 1 teaspoon roasted garlic paste
- 1 teaspoon ancho chili powder
- 1/2 teaspoon dried basil
- 1/2 teaspoon dried Mexican oregano
- 1/4 teaspoon freshly ground black pepper, or more to taste
- Sea salt, to taste
- 10 ounces Ricotta cheese, at room temperature
- 1 cup Mexican cheese,shredded
- 1 cup broth, preferably homemade
- 2 ripe tomatoes, chopped
- 1/3 cup salsa verde

Directions

1. Press the "Sauté" button to heat up your Instant Pot. Once hot, heat the sesame oil; now, sauté the onion until translucent.
2. Stir in ground turkey and continue to sauté until it is no longer pink. Add the remaining ingredients and stir until everything is combined well.
3. Secure the lid. Choose "Manual" mode and High pressure; cook for 6 minutes. Once cooking is complete, use a natural pressure release; carefully remove the lid. Bon appétit!

Meatballs with Cheese

Preparation Time: 15 minutes

Servings 8

Nutritional Values per serving: 277 Calories; 17.4g Fat; 3.1g Total Carbs; 25.8g Protein; 0.9g Sugars

Ingredients

- 1 pound ground beef
- 1/2 cup pork chicharron, crushed
- 1/2 cup Parmesan cheese, grated
- 2 eggs, beaten
- 2 tablespoons fresh scallions, chopped
- 2 tablespoons fresh cilantro, chopped
- 1 teaspoon garlic, minced
- Sea salt, to your liking
- 1/2 teaspoon ground black pepper
- 1/2 teaspoon cayenne pepper
- 1 cup Colby cheese, cubed
- 2 teaspoons olive oil
- 1/2 cup chicken broth
- 1/2 cup BBQ sauce

Directions

1. In a mixing dish, thoroughly combine ground beef, pork chicharron,Parmesan cheese, eggs, scallions, cilantro, garlic, salt, black pepper, and cayenne pepper; mix until everything is well incorporated.
2. Now, shape the mixture into balls. Press one cheese cube into center of each meatball, sealing it inside.
3. Press the "Sauté" button and heat the olive oil. Sear the meatballs for a couple of minutes or until browned on all sides. Pour in chicken broth and BBQ sauce.
4. Secure the lid. Choose the "Manual" setting and cook for 8 minutes under High pressure. Once cooking is complete, use a quick pressure release; carefully remove the lid.
5. Serve your meatballs with the sauce. Bon appétit!

Spanish Fat Bombs

Preparation Time: 10 minutes

Servings 8

Nutritional Values per serving: 307 Calories; 26.8g Fat; 5.1g Total Carbs; 10.9g Protein; 2.9g Sugars

Ingredients

- 1 tablespoon tallow, melted
- 1 yellow onion, chopped
- 1 pound Chorizo sausage
- 1 garlic clove, minced
- 1 red bell pepper, chopped
- 1 cup chicken broth
- 1/2 teaspoon deli mustard
- 1 plum tomato, puréed
- 10 ounces Halloumi cheese, crumbled
- 1/3 cup mayonnaise

Directions

1. Press the "Sauté" button and melt the tallow. Once hot, cook the onion until tender and translucent.
2. Add Chorizo and garlic to your Instant Pot; cook until the sausage is no longer pink; crumble the sausage with a fork.
3. Now, stir in bell pepper, broth, mustard, and tomato.
4. Secure the lid. Choose "Manual" mode and High pressure; cook for 4 minutes. Once cooking is complete, use a quick pressure release; carefully remove the lid.
5. Add the cheese and mayo. Shape the mixture into 2-inch balls and serve. Bon appétit!

Yummy Cocktail Wieners

Preparation Time: 10 minutes

Servings 10

Nutritional Values per serving: 257 Calories; 22.7g Fat; 1.4g Total Carbs; 10.8g Protein; 0.2g Sugars

Ingredients

- 1 pound cocktail wieners
- 1/2 pound sliced bacon, cold cut into slices
- 1/2 cup chicken broth
- 1/2 cup water
- 1/4 cup low-carb ketchup
- 2 tablespoons apple cider vinegar
- 1 tablespoon onion powder
- 1 tablespoon ground mustard
- Salt and pepper to taste

Directions

1. Wrap each cocktail wiener with a slice of bacon; secure with a toothpick.
2. Then, place one layer of bacon wrapped cocktail wieners in the bottom of the Instant Pot. Repeat layering until you run out of the cocktail wieners.
3. In a mixing bowl, thoroughly combine the remaining ingredients. Pour this mixture over the bacon wrapped cocktail wieners.
4. Secure the lid. Choose "Manual" mode and Low pressure; cook for 3 minutes. Once cooking is complete, use a natural pressure release; carefully remove the lid. Enjoy!

Fresh Brussels Sprouts with Aioli Sauce

Preparation Time: 10 minutes

Servings 4

Nutritional Values per serving: 161 Calories; 13.4g Fat; 6g Total Carbs; 3.1g Protein; 2.5g Sugars

Ingredients

- 1 tablespoon butter
- 1/2 cup scallions, chopped
- 3/4 pound Brussels sprouts
- Aioli Sauce:
- 1/4 cup mayonnaise
- 1 garlic clove, minced
- 1 tablespoon fresh lemon juice
- 1/2 teaspoon Dijon mustard

Directions

1. Press the "Sauté" button and melt the butter. Once hot, cook the scallions until softened. Now, add Brussels sprouts and sauté them for 1 minute more.
2. Secure the lid. Choose "Manual" mode and High pressure; cook for 4 minutes. Once cooking is complete, use a quick pressure release; carefully remove the lid.
3. Meanwhile, mix mayonnaise, garlic, lemon juice, Dijon mustard. Serve Brussels sprouts with Aioli sauce on the side. Bon appétit!

Cheesy Bacon Bites

Preparation Time: 10 minutes

Servings 8

Nutritional Values per serving: 187 Calories; 14.2g Fat; 5.2g Total Carbs; 9.4g Protein; 3.4g Sugars

Ingredients

- 1/2 pound rutabaga, grated
- 4 slices meaty bacon, chopped
- 7 ounces Gruyère cheese, shredded
- 3 eggs, beaten
- 3 tablespoons almond flour
- 1 teaspoon granulated garlic
- 1 teaspoon shallot powder
- Sea salt and ground black pepper, to taste

Directions

1. Add 1 cup of water and a metal trivet to the Instant Pot.
2. Mix all of the above ingredients until everything is well incorporated.
3. Put the mixture into a silicone pod tray that is previously greased with a nonstick cooking spray. Cover the tray with a sheet of aluminum foil and lower it onto the trivet.
4. Secure the lid. Choose “Manual” mode and Low pressure; cook for 5 minutes. Once cooking is complete, use a quick pressure release; carefully remove the lid. Bon appétit!

Juicy Meatballs

Preparation Time: 25 MIN

Serving: 8

Ingredients:

- 1 pound grass-fed ground chicken
- 1 organic egg
- 1/3 cup almond flour
- ½ tsp garlic powder
- Salt and freshly ground black pepper, to taste
- ¾ cup hot sauce
- 2 tbsp. olive oil
- 2 tbsp. melted butter
- ½ cup blue cheese dressing

Directions:

1. In a bowl, add all ingredients except, oil, hot sauce, butter and blue cheese dressing and mix until well combined.
2. Make equal sized meatballs from the mixture.
3. Place the oil in the Instant Pot and select "Sauté". Then add the meatballs and cook for about 4-5 minutes or until browned from all sides.

4. Meanwhile, in a bowl, mix together hot sauce and butter.
5. Select the "Cancel" and place butter mixture over meatballs.
6. Secure the lid and place the pressure valve to "Seal" position.
7. Select the "Poultry" and just use the default time of 5 minutes.
8. Select the "Cancel" and carefully do a Quick release.
9. Remove the lid and serve immediately with the topping of dressing.

Nutritional Values per serving:

Calories 278

Total Fat 21.6g

Net Carbs 0.33g

Protein 19g

Fiber 0.6g

Perfect Chicken Wings

Preparation Time: 40 MIN

Serving: 4

Ingredients:

- 1½ pounds grass-fed chicken wings
- ¼ cup sugar-free tomato puree
- 2-3 drops liquid stevia
- 1 tbsp. fresh lemon juice
- Salt and freshly ground black pepper, to taste

Directions:

1. In the bottom of Instant Pot, arrange a steamer trivet and pour 1 cup of water.
2. Place the pan on top of the trivet.
3. Place chicken wings on top of the trivet, standing vertically.
4. Secure the lid and place the pressure valve to "Seal" position.
5. Select "Manual" and cook under "High Pressure" for about 10 minutes.
6. Preheat the oven to broiler.
7. Select the "Cancel" and carefully do a Quick release.
8. Meanwhile, in a bowl, add remaining ingredients and beat until well combined.

9. Remove the lid and transfer chicken wings to the bowl of sauce.
10. Coat the wings with sauce generously.
11. Arrange the chicken wings onto a parchment paper lined baking sheet and broil for about 5 minutes.
12. Serve hot with remaining sauce.

Nutritional Values per serving:

Calories 330

Total Fat 12.7g

Net Carbs 0.37g

Protein 49.5g

Fiber 0.3g

2-Ingredients Chicken Wings

Preparation Time: 40 MIN

Serving: 6

Ingredients:

- 2 pounds grass-fed chicken wings and drumettes
- ½ cup sugar-free BBQ sauce

Directions:

1. In the bottom of Instant Pot, arrange a steamer basket and pour 1 cup of water.
2. Place the wings and drumettes into the steamer basket.
3. Secure the lid and place the pressure valve to "Seal" position.
4. Select "Manual" and cook under "High Pressure" for about 5 minutes.
5. Preheat the oven to 450 degrees F. Arrange a wire rack on a baking sheet.
6. Select the "Cancel" and carefully do a Natural release.
7. Remove the lid and transfer wings and drumettes to a large plate.
8. With paper towels, pat dry the wings and drumettes.
9. In a bowl, add wings and drumettes with BBQ sauce and toss to coat well.

10. Place the wings and drumettes onto the prepared baking sheet in a single layer.
11. Bake for about 8-15 minutes.
12. Remove from oven and serve warm.

Nutritional Values per serving:

Calories 319

Total Fat 11.3g

Net Carbs 1.26g

Protein 43.7g

Fiber 0.1g

Sticky Chicken Wings

Preparation Time: 40 MIN

Serving: 8

Ingredients:

- 3 pounds drum and wings separated grass-fed chicken wings
- 6 tbsp. olive oil (divided
- 1 cup sugar-free teriyaki sauce
- 1 tbsp. fresh lemon juice
- 1 tbsp. Erythritol
- ½ tsp crushed red pepper flakes

Directions:

1. In a large bowl, add chicken wings, 4 tablespoons of oil, teriyaki sauce, lemon juice and Erythritol and mix well.
2. Refrigerate for at least 2 hours.
3. Remove chicken wings from the bowl, reserving marinade.
4. Place the remaining oil in the Instant Pot and select "Sauté". Then add the wings and cook for about -4 minutes or until browned from all sides.
5. Select the "Cancel" and place reserved marinade over wings evenly.

6. Secure the lid and place the pressure valve to "Seal" position.
7. Select "Manual" and cook under "High Pressure" for about 7 minutes.
8. Preheat the oven to broiler.
9. Select the "Cancel" and carefully do a "Natural" release for about 10 minutes and then do a "Quick" release.
10. Remove the lid and transfer the wings onto a baking sheet in a single layer.
11. Broil for about 6-8 minutes.
12. Remove from oven and serve warm with the sprinkling of red pepper flakes.

Nutritional Values per serving:

Calories 446

Total Fat 23.2g

Net Carbs 0.95g

Protein 51.4g

Fiber 0.1g

Simple Boiled Peanuts

Preparation Time: 1½ HOUR

Serving: 6

Ingredients:

1 pound raw peanuts in the shell

1/3 cup coarse sea salt

Filtered water, as required

Directions:

1. Rinse the peanuts under cold running water and remove any twigs and roots.
2. In the bottom of Instant Pot, place peanuts, salt and enough water to cover the peanuts and stir.
3. Place a plate or trivet on top of peanuts.
4. Secure the lid and place the pressure valve to "Seal" position.
5. Select "Manual" and cook under "High Pressure" for about 80 minutes.
6. Select the "Cancel" and carefully do a "Natural" release.
7. Remove the lid and keep aside to cool.
8. Drain well and serve.

Nutritional Values per serving:

Calories 429

Total Fat 37.2g

Net Carbs 2.03g

Protein 19.5g

Fiber 6.4g

Southern Boiled Peanuts

Preparation Time: 1 HOUR 40 MIN

Serving: 6

Ingredients:

- 1 pound jumbo raw peanuts
- ½ cup sea salt
- 1 tbsp. Cajun seasoning
- Filtered water, as required

Directions:

1. Rinse the peanuts under cold running water and remove any twigs and roots.
2. In the bottom of Instant Pot, place peanuts, salt, Cajun seasoning and enough water to cover the peanuts and stir.
3. Place a plate or trivet on top of peanuts.
4. Secure the lid and place the pressure valve to "Seal" position.
5. Select "Manual" and cook under "High Pressure" for about 65-90 minutes.
6. Select the "Cancel" and carefully do a "Natural" release.
7. Remove the lid and keep aside to cool.
8. Drain well and serve.

Nutritional Values per serving:

Calories 429

Total Fat 37.2g

Net Carbs 2.03g

Protein 19.5g

Fiber 6.4g

Hard Boiled Eggs

Preparation Time: 10 MIN

Serving: 4

Ingredients:

- 8 large Eggs
- 1 cup Water

Instructions:

1. Set the wire rack in the Instant Pot and pour in the water.
2. Carefully place eggs in and place and lock the lid.
3. Manually set the cooking time to 4 minutes at high pressure.
4. Quick release the pressure and transfer the eggs in iced water for 5 minutes for easier peeling.
5. Use immediately or store in the fridge for later use.

Nutritional Values per serving:

Calories: 156

Total Fats: 10.6g

Net Carbs: 1.1g

Proteins: 12.6g

Fibers: 0g

Steamed Artichokes

Preparation Time: 20 MIN

Serving: 4

Ingredients:

- 4 medium Artichokes
- 1 wedge Lemon
- 1 cup Water

Directions:

1. Wash the artichokes well and with a knife cut off the stem and around an inch of the top.
2. Rub the cut on top with the lemon, to prevent browning, and gently spread the leaves a bit.
3. Place the artichokes in a steamer insert in the Instant Pot and pour in a cup of water.
4. Place and lock the lid, and set the Instant Pot manual to 10 minutes cooking time at high pressure.
5. When done let the Instant Pot naturally release the pressure for 10 minutes and then open the valve for quick release.
6. Serve warm with a dipping sauce.

Nutritional Values per serving:

Calories: 60

Total Fats: 0.2g

Net Carbs: 6.6g

Proteins: 4.2g

Fibers: 6.9g

Zingy Boiled Peanuts

Preparation Time: 1 HOUR 40 MIN

Serving: 6

Ingredients:

- 1 pound raw peanuts
- 1/3 cup Old Bay seasoning
- ¼ cup kosher salt
- ¼ cup apple cider vinegar
- 1 tbsp. mustard seeds
- 1 bay leaf
- Filtered water, as required

Directions:

1. Rinse the peanuts under cold running water and remove any twigs and roots.
2. In the bottom of Instant Pot, add all ingredients and enough water to cover the peanuts and stir.
3. Place a plate or trivet on top of peanuts.
4. Secure the lid and place the pressure valve to "Seal" position.
5. Select "Manual" and cook under "High Pressure" for about 75-90 minutes.
6. Select the "Cancel" and carefully do a "Natural" release.
7. Remove the lid and keep aside to cool.

8. Drain well and serve.

Nutritional Values per serving:

Calories 4540

Total Fat 37.8g

Net Carbs 0.48g

Protein 20g

Fiber 6.7g

Unique Party Food

Preparation Time: 18 MIN

Serving: 4

Ingredients:

- 1 pound asparagus spears
- 8-ounce sliced prosciutto

Directions:

1. Wrap the prosciutto slices around asparagus spears.
2. In the bottom of Instant Pot, arrange a steamer basket and pour 2 cups of water.
3. Place the carrots into the steamer basket.
4. Arrange any extra un-wrapped spears in the bottom of the steamer basket in a single layer.
5. Place prosciutto-wrapped asparagus on top in a single layer.
6. Secure the lid and place the pressure valve to "Seal" position.
7. Select "Manual" and cook under "High Pressure" for about 2-3 minutes.
8. Select the "Cancel" and carefully do a Natural release.
9. Remove the lid and serve warm

Nutritional Values per serving:

Calories 105

Total Fat 3.3g

Net Carbs 1.32 g

Protein 14.4g

Fiber 2,1g

Decadent Liver Pâté

Preparation Time: 25 MIN

Serving: 6

Ingredients:

- 1 tsp olive oil
- 1 roughly chopped medium yellow onion
- Salt and freshly ground black pepper, to taste
- ¾ pound grass-fed chicken livers
- 1 bay leaf
- ¼ cup homemade chicken broth
- 1 tbsp. fresh lemon juice
- 2 anchovies in oil
- 1 tbsp. capers
- 1 tbsp. butter

Directions:

1. Place the oil in the Instant Pot and select "Sauté". Then add the onion with a little salt and black pepper and cook for about 2-3 minutes.
2. Add the chicken livers and bay leaf and cook for about 2 minutes.
3. Add the broth and scrape brown bits from the bottom.
4. Select the "Cancel" and stir the mixture once.

5. Secure the lid and place the pressure valve to "Seal" position.
6. Select "Manual" and cook under "High Pressure" for about 5 minutes.
7. Select the "Cancel" and carefully do a Natural release.
8. Remove the lid and discard the bay leaf.
9. Stir in anchovies and capers and with a stick blender, blend the mixture until pureed.
10. Stir in butter and rum and transfer to a bowl.
11. Refrigerate to chill before serving.

Nutritional Values per serving:

Calories 142

Total Fat 7.3g

Net Carbs 0.4g

Protein 15.7g

Fiber 0.5g

Exotic Mushroom Pâté

Preparation Time: 25 MIN

Serving: 6

Ingredients:

- 1 cup boiling water
- ¾ cup rinsed dry porcini mushrooms
- 2 tbsp. unsalted butter
- 1 sliced small yellow onion
- 1 pound thinly sliced fresh cremini mushrooms
- 2-3 tbsp. homemade chicken broth
- 1 tbsp. fresh lemon juice
- 1 bay leaf
- Salt and ground white pepper, to taste
- 1 tbsp. extra-virgin olive oil
- 3 tbsp. finely grated Parmigiana Reggiano cheese

Directions:

1. In a heat-proof bowl, mix together boiling water and dry porcini mushrooms.
2. Cover the bowl tightly and keep aside.
3. Place the butter in the Instant Pot and select "Sauté". Then add the onion and cook for about 5 minutes.
4. Add the fresh mushrooms and cook for about 5 minutes.

5. Add broth and lemon juice and cook for about 5 minutes or until all the liquid is absorbed.
6. Select the "Cancel" and stir in porcini mushrooms and with soaking liquid, bay leaf, salt and black pepper.
7. Secure the lid and place the pressure valve to "Seal" position.
8. Select "Manual" and cook under "High Pressure" for about 12 minutes.
9. Select the "Cancel" and carefully do a Natural release.
10. Remove the lid and discard the bay leaf.
11. Add the olive oil and with an immersion blender, blend the mixture until smooth.
12. Add the cheese and blend until well combined.
13. Transfer the mixture to a bowl and refrigerate for about 2 hours before serving.

Nutritional Values per serving:

Calories 115

Total Fat 6.6g

Net Carbs 0.96g

Protein 6.3g

Fiber 0.7g

Garden Fresh Salsa

Preparation Time: 30 MIN

Serving: 20

Ingredients:

- 4 cups cored, peeled and chopped tomatoes
- 1 (15-ouncecan sugar-free tomato sauce
- 1 (6-ouncecan sugar-free tomato paste
- 1 chopped medium yellow onion
- 2 seeded and chopped large green bell peppers
- 3 seeded and chopped jalapeño peppers
- 4 minced garlic cloves
- ½ cup apple cider vinegar
- 1 tbsp. hot sauce
- 1 tbsp. ground cumin
- Kosher salt, to taste

Directions:

1. In the bottom of Instant Pot, place all ingredients and stir to combine.
2. Secure the lid and place the pressure valve to "Seal" position.
3. Select "Manual" and cook under "High Pressure" for about 15 minutes.
4. Select the "Cancel" and carefully do a "Natural" release.

5. Remove the lid and keep aside to cool for about 20 minutes.
6. Transfer the salsa into wide mouth pint jars and seal with lids.
7. Refrigerate to chill before serving.

Nutritional Values per serving:

Calories 29

Total Fat 0.3g

Net Carbs 0.30g

Protein 1.3g

Fiber 1.5g

Party Meatballs

Preparation Time: 40 MIN

Serving: 8

Ingredients:

- 1 pound lean ground turkey
- 1 organic egg
- ¼ tsp dried thyme
- ¼ tsp dried oregano
- ¼ tsp dried rosemary
- ¼ tsp garlic powder
- Salt and freshly ground black pepper, to taste
- 1½ cups sugar-free tomato sauce

Directions:

1. In a bowl, add all ingredients except tomato sauce and mix until well combined.
2. Make equal sized meatballs from the mixture.
3. In the bottom of Instant Pot, place meatballs and tomato sauce and gently stir to combine.
4. Secure the lid and place the pressure valve to "Seal" position.
5. Select "Manual" and cook under "High Pressure" for about 25 minutes.
6. Select the "Cancel" and carefully do a "Quick" release.

7. Remove the lid and serve.

Nutritional Values per serving:

Calories 101

Total Fat 4.7g

Net Carbs 0.18g

Protein 12.5g

Fiber 0.8g

Cheese Loaded Burgers

Preparation Time: 20 MIN

Serving: 2

Ingredients:

- 1 pound grass-fed lean ground beef
- 1 tbsp. Worcestershire sauce
- ¼ tsp garlic powder
- Salt and freshly ground black pepper, to taste
- 2-ounce shredded cheddar cheese

Directions:

1. In a large bowl, add ground beef, Worcestershire Sauce, garlic powder, salt and black pepper and mix until well combined.
2. Make 4 equal sized balls from the mixture.
3. With your hands, flatten each ball.
4. Place 1-ounce cheese in the center of 2 of the flattened balls.
5. Cover each with remaining 2 flatten balls, pressing the edges together well.
6. In the bottom of Instant Pot, arrange a steamer tray and pour ½ cup of water.
7. Place burgers on top of steamer tray.

8. Secure the lid and place the pressure valve to "Seal" position.
9. Select "Manual" and cook under "High Pressure" for about 5 minutes.
10. Select the "Cancel" and carefully do a "Natural" release.
11. Remove the lid and serve.

Nutritional Values per serving:

Calories 544

Total Fat 23.5g

Net Carbs 1g

Protein 75.9g

Fiber 0g

Mini Sausage Bites

Preparation Time: 20 MIN

Serving: 10

Ingredients:

- 2 pounds gluten-free cut into 1/3-inch thick slices Kielbasa links
- 1 cup sugar-free BBQ sauce
- ½ cup filtered water

Directions:

1. In the bottom of Instant Pot, place all ingredients and stir to combine.
2. Secure the lid and place the pressure valve to "Seal" position.
3. Select "Manual" and cook under "High Pressure" for about 5 minutes.
4. Select the "Cancel" and carefully do a "Natural" release for about 10 minutes and then do a "Quick" release.
5. Remove the lid and transfer the mixture to a serving bowl.
6. Keep aside for about 10-15 minutes before serving.

Nutritional Values per serving:

Calories 243

Total Fat 16g

Net Carbs 1.26g

Protein 11.9g

Fiber 0.2g

Refreshing Curd

Preparation time: 10 minutes

Cooking time: 5 minutes

Servings: 4

Ingredients:

- 3 tablespoons stevia
- 12 ounces raspberries
- 2 egg yolks
- 2 tablespoons lemon juice
- 2 tablespoons ghee

Directions:

1. Put raspberries in your instant pot, add stevia and lemon juice, stir, cover and cook on High for 2 minutes.
2. Strain this into a bowl, add egg yolks, stir well and return to your pot.
3. Set the pot on Simmer mode, cook for 2 minutes, add ghee, stir well, transfer to a container and serve cold.
4. Enjoy!

Nutritional Values per serving: Calories 132, fat 1, fiber 0, carbs 2, protein 4

The Best Jam Ever

Preparation time: 10 minutes

Cooking time: 5 minutes

Servings: 6

Ingredients:

- 4 and ½ cups peaches, peeled and cubed
- 4 tablespoons stevia
- ¼ cup crystallized ginger, chopped

Directions:

1. Set your instant pot on Simmer mode, add peaches, ginger and stevia, stir, bring to a boil, cover and cook on High for 5 minutes.
2. Divide into bowls and serve cold.
3. Enjoy!

Nutritional Values per serving: Calories 53, fat 0, fiber 0, carbs 0, protein 2

Divine Pears

Preparation time: 10 minutes

Cooking time: 4 minutes

Servings: 12

Ingredients:

- 8 pears, cored and cut into quarters
- 1 teaspoon cinnamon powder
- 2 apples, peeled, cored and cut into quarters
- ¼ cup natural apple juice

Directions:

1. In your instant pot, mix pears with apples, cinnamon and apple juice, stir, cover and cook on High for 4 minutes.
2. Blend using an immersion blender, divide into small jars and serve cold
3. Enjoy!

Nutritional Values per serving: Calories 100, fat 0, fiber 0, carbs 0, protein 2

Berry Marmalade

Preparation time: 10 minutes

Cooking time: 20 minutes

Servings: 12

Ingredients:

- 1 pound cranberries
- 1 pound strawberries
- ½ pound blueberries
- ounces black currant
- 4 tablespoons stevia
- Zest from 1 lemon
- A pinch of salt
- 2 tablespoon water

Directions:

1. In your instant pot, mix strawberries with cranberries, blueberries, currants, lemon zest, stevia and water, stir, cover and cook on High for 10 minutes.
2. Divide into jars and serve cold.
3. Enjoy!

Nutritional Values per serving: Calories 87, fat 2, fiber 0, carbs 1, protein 2

Orange Delight

Preparation time: 10 minutes

Cooking time: 25 minutes

Servings: 8

Ingredients:

- Juice from 2 lemons
- 6 tablespoons stevia
- 1 pound oranges, peeled and halved
- 1-pint water

Directions:

1. In your instant pot, mix lemon juice with orange juice and orange segments, water and stevia, cover and cook on High for 15 minutes.
2. Divide into jars and serve cold.

Nutritional Values per serving: Calories 75, fat 0, fiber 0, carbs 2, protein 2

Simple Squash Pie

Preparation time: 10 minutes

Cooking time: 14 minutes

Serving: 8

Ingredients:

- 2 pounds butternut squash, peeled and chopped
- 2 eggs
- 2 cups water
- 1 cup coconut milk
- 2 tablespoons honey
- 1 teaspoon cinnamon powder
- ½ teaspoon ginger powder
- ¼ teaspoon cloves, ground
- 1 tablespoon arrowroot powder
- Chopped pecans

Directions:

1. Put 1 cup water in your instant pot, add the steamer basket, add squash pieces, cover, cook on High for 4 minutes, drain, transfer to a bowl and mash.
2. Add honey, milk, eggs, cinnamon, ginger and cloves, stir very well and pour into ramekins.
3. Add the rest of the water to your instant pot, add the steamer basket, add ramekins inside, cover and cook on High for 10 minutes.
4. Garnish with chopped pecans and serve.
5. Enjoy!

Nutritional Values per serving: Calories 132, fat 1, fiber 2, carbs 2, protein 3

Winter Pudding

Preparation time: 10 minutes

Cooking time: 40 minutes

Servings: 4

Ingredients:

- 4 ounces dried cranberries, soaked for a few hours and drained
- 2 cups water
- 4 ounces apricots, chopped
- 1 cup coconut flour
- 3 teaspoons baking powder
- 3 tablespoons stevia
- 1 teaspoon ginger powder
- A pinch of cinnamon powder
- 15 tablespoons ghee
- 3 tablespoons maple syrup
- 4 eggs
- 1 carrot, grated

Directions:

1. In a blender, mix flour with baking powder, stevia, cinnamon and ginger and pulse a few times.
2. Add ghee, maple syrup, eggs, carrots, cranberries and apricots, stir and spread into a greased pudding pan.
3. Add the water to your instant pot, add the steamer basket, add the pudding, cover and cook on High for 30 minutes.
4. Leave pudding to cool down before serving.
5. Enjoy!

Nutritional Values per serving: Calories 213, fat 2, fiber 1, carbs 3, protein 3

Banana Dessert

Preparation time: 10 minutes

Cooking time: 30 minutes

Servings: 6

Ingredients:

- 2 tablespoons stevia
- 1/3 cup ghee, soft
- 1 teaspoon vanilla
- 1 egg
- 2 bananas, mashed
- 1 teaspoon baking powder
- 1 and ½ cups coconut flour
- ½ teaspoons baking soda
- 1/3 cup coconut milk
- 2 cups water
- Cooking spray

Directions:

1. In a bowl, mix milk stevia, ghee, egg, vanilla and bananas and stir everything.
2. In another bowl, mix flour with salt, baking powder and soda.
3. Combine the 2 mixtures, stir well and pour into a greased cake pan.
4. Add the water to your pot, add the steamer basket, add the cake pan, cover and cook at High for 30 minutes.
5. Leave cake to cool down, slice and serve.
6. Enjoy!

Nutritional Values per serving: Calories 243, fat 1, fiber 1, carbs 2, protein 4

Apple Cake

Preparation time: 10 minutes

Cooking time: 1 hour and 10 minutes

Servings: 6

Ingredients:

- 3 cups apples, cored and cubed
- 1 cup water
- 3 tablespoons stevia
- 1 tablespoon vanilla
- 2 eggs
- 1 tablespoon apple pie spice
- 2 cups coconut flour
- 1 tablespoon baking powder
- 1 tablespoon ghee

Directions:

1. In a bowl mix eggs with ghee, apple pie spice, vanilla, apples and stevia and stir using your mixer.
2. In another bowl, mix baking powder with flour, stir, add to apple mix, stir again well and transfer to a cake pan.
3. Add 1 cup water to your instant pot, add the steamer basket, add cake pan, cover and cook at High for 1 hour and 10 minutes.
4. Cool cake down, slice and serve it.
5. Enjoy!

Nutritional Values per serving: Calories 100, fat 2, fiber 1, carbs 2, protein 2

Special Vanilla Dessert

Preparation time: 10 minutes

Cooking time: 10 minutes

Servings: 4

Ingredients:

- 1 cup almond milk
- 4 tablespoons flax meal
- 2 tablespoons coconut flour
- 2 and ½ cups water
- 2 tablespoons stevia
- 1 teaspoon espresso powder
- 2 teaspoons vanilla extract
- Coconut cream for serving

Directions:

1. In your instant pot, mix flax meal with flour, water, stevia, milk and espresso powder, stir, cover and cook on high for 10 minutes.
2. Add vanilla extract, stir well, leave aside for 5 minutes, divide into bowls and serve with coconut cream on top.
3. Enjoy!

Nutritional Values per serving: Calories 182, fat 2, fiber 1, carbs 3, protein 4

Tasty and Amazing Pear Dessert

Preparation time: 10 minutes

Cooking time: 6 minutes

Servings: 4

Ingredients:

- 1 cup water
- 2 cups pear, peeled and cubed
- 2 cups coconut milk
- 1 tablespoon ghee
- ¼ cups brown stevia
- ½ teaspoon cinnamon powder
- 4 tablespoons flax meal
- ½ cup walnuts, chopped
- ½ cup raisins

Directions:

1. In a heat proof dish, mix milk with stevia, ghee, flax meal, cinnamon, raisins, pears and walnuts and stir.
2. Put the water in your instant pot, add the steamer basket, place heat proof dish inside, cover and cook on High for 6 minutes.
3. Divide this great dessert into small cups and serve cold.
4. Enjoy!

Nutritional Values per serving: Calories 162, fat 3, fiber 1, carbs 2, protein 6

Cranberries Jam

Preparation time: 10 minutes

Cooking time: 15 minutes

Servings: 12

Ingredients:

- 16 ounces cranberries
- 4 ounces raisins
- 3 ounces water+ ¼ cup water
- 8 ounces figs
- 16 ounces strawberries, chopped
- Zest from 1 lemon

Directions:

1. Put figs in your blender, add ¼ cup water, pulse well and strain into a bowl.
2. In your instant pot, mix strawberries with cranberries, lemon zest, raisins, 3 ounces water and figs puree, stir, cover the pot, cook at High for 15 minutes, divide into small jars and serve.

Nutritional Values per serving: Calories 73, fat 1, fiber 1, carbs 2, protein 3

Lemon Jam

Preparation time: 10 minutes

Cooking time: 12 minutes

Servings: 8

Ingredients:

- 2 pounds lemons, sliced
- 2 cups dates
- 1 cup water
- 1 tablespoon vinegar

Directions:

1. Put dates in your blender, add water and pulse really well.
2. Put lemon slices in your instant pot, add dates paste and vinegar, stir, cover and cook on High for 12 minutes.
3. Stir, divide into small jars and serve.
4. Enjoy!

Nutritional Values per serving: Calories 72, fat 2, fiber 1, carbs 2, protein 6

Special Dessert

Preparation time: 10 minutes

Cooking time: 25 minutes

Servings: 4

Ingredients:

- 3 cups rooibos tea
- 1 tablespoon cinnamon, ground
- 2 cups cauliflower, riced
- 2 apples, diced
- 1 teaspoon cloves, ground
- 1 teaspoon turmeric, ground
- A drizzle of honey

Directions:

1. Put cauliflower rice in your instant pot, add tea, stir, cover and cook at High for 10 minutes
2. Add cinnamon, apples, turmeric and cloves, stir, cover and cook at High for 10 minutes mode.
3. Divide into bowls, drizzle honey on top and serve.
4. Enjoy!

Nutritional Values per serving: Calories 152, fat 2, fiber 1, carbs 5, protein 6

Spicy Cannellini Bean Salad with Dates

Ready in: 35 minutes + chilling time

Serving: 12

Nutritional Values per serving: Calories 195; Carbs 29g; Fat 3g; Protein 9g

Ingredients

- 1 cup dry Cannellini Beans, soaked
- 1 cup fresh Dates, halved, pitted
- 2 ½ cups frozen Green peas, thawed
- 1 cup Scallions, chopped
- 1 cup Tomatoes, thinly sliced
- 3 Cloves Garlic, minced
- 1 tbsp Olive Oil
- ¼ cup White Wine Vinegar
- ¼ cup Tamari Sauce
- 2 tsp Chili Paste
- Salt and Black Pepper, to taste
- ½ tsp Red Pepper flakes, for garnish

Directions

1. To prepare the dressing, whisk tamari sauce, oil, vinegar, chili paste and garlic. Refrigerate overnight.
2. Place the beans in your pressure cooker and pour water to cover them. Seal the lid and switch the pressure release valve to close. Select BEANS/CHILI mode and cook for 25 minutes at High Pressure.

3. Once the cooking is complete, do a quick pressure release. Drain the beans and transfer to a serving bowl. Add in the rest of the ingredients, and toss with the dressing until well coated.

Savory Vegetarian Sandwiches

Preparation Time: 35 minutes

Serving: 4

Nutritional Values per serving: Calories 488; Carbs 62g; Fat 19g; Protein 28g

Ingredients

- 1 tbsp Vegetable Oil
- 4 Vegetarian Sausages, sliced
- 1 Garlic Cloves, crushed
- ½ cup Tamari Sauce
- 2 Shallots, chopped
- 2 cups roasted Vegetable Stock
- 2 Bell Peppers, deveined and sliced
- 4 Burger Buns
- 1 cup freshly grated Cheddar Cheese
- Salt and ground Black Pepper, to taste
- 2 ½ cups Water

Directions

1. Heat oil on SAUTÉ at High and cook the garlic and shallots, until tender, for about 3 minutes. Stir in the sausages and cook for another 5 minutes. Add in the remaining ingredients, except for the buns and cheese.
2. Select PRESSURE COOK/MANUAL and cook for 15 minutes at High. Once ready, do a quick pressure

release. Preheat oven to 460 degrees F. Divide prepared mixture among 4 burger buns and top with grated cheese.

3. Bake the sandwiches in the oven for 6-7 minutes, or until the cheese melts. Serve immediately!

Eat-me" Squash and Sweet Potato Creamy Soup

Preparation Time: 30 minutes

Serving: 4

Nutritional Values per serving: Calories 243; Carbs 33g; Fat 9g; Protein 7g

Ingredients

- 2 cups Squash, cubed
- 2 cups Sweet Potatoes, cubed
- 2 tbsp Olive Oil
- 1 Onion, diced
- 1 tbsp Heavy Cream
- 3 cups Veggie Broth
- A pinch of Thyme

Directions

1. On SAUTÉ at High, warm the oil, and add the onions. Cook until soft, about 3 minutes. Stir in the potatoes and squash and cook for an additional minute, or until they begin to 'sweat'.
2. Pour the broth over and stir in the thyme. Seal the lid, choose BEANS/CHILI for 10 minutes at High. When done, do a natural pressure release, for about 10 minutes. Stir in the cream, and serve.

Green Pea Medley

Preparation Time: 25 minutes

Servings 6

Nutritional Values per serving: 173 Calories; 6.6g Fat; 22.7g Carbs; 7.7g Protein; 7.9g Sugars

Ingredients

- 2 tablespoons canola oil
- 1 teaspoon cumin seeds
- 2 ½ cups green peas, whole
- 2 ripe Roma tomatoes, seeded and crushed
- 3 cups roasted vegetable stock
- 1 shallot, diced
- 2 cloves garlic, minced
- 2 carrots, chopped
- 2 parsnips, chopped
- 1 red bell pepper, seeded and chopped
- 2 bay leaves
- Sea salt and ground black pepper, to taste
- 1 teaspoon cayenne pepper
- 1/2 teaspoon dried dill

Directions

1. Press the "Sauté" button to preheat the Instant Pot. Once hot, add the oil. Then, sauté the cumin seeds for 30 seconds.
2. Add shallot, garlic, carrots, parsnip and pepper; continue to sauté for 3 to 4 minutes more or until vegetables are tender.
3. Now, stir in the remaining ingredients.
4. Secure the lid. Choose the "Manual" mode and cook for 18 minutes under High pressure. Once cooking is complete, use a natural release; carefully remove the lid.
5. Serve with cream cheese if desired. Bon appétit!

Spicy Veggie and Adzuki Bean Soup

Preparation Time: 30 minutes

Servings 4

Nutritional Values per serving: 474 Calories; 7.6g Fat; 84g Carbs; 20.5g Protein; 7.8g Sugars

Ingredients

- 2 tablespoons olive oil
- 2 onions, chopped
- 2 carrots chopped
- 2 parsnips, chopped
- 1 celery with leaves, chopped
- 2 Yukon gold potatoes, peeled and diced
- 2 ripe tomatoes, pureed
- 12 ounces Adzuki brans, soaked overnight
- 1 teaspoon cayenne pepper
- 1 teaspoon dried basil
- 1/2 teaspoon marjoram
- 1 teaspoon black garlic powder
- 1 teaspoon dried chive flakes
- A few drops Sriracha
- Kosher salt and ground black pepper, to taste
- 4 cups boiling water

Directions

1. Press the “Sauté” button to heat up the Instant Pot. Now, heat the olive oil and sweat the onions until just tender.
2. Add the other ingredients; stir to combine well. Secure the lid and choose the “Manual” mode. Cook for 10 minutes at High Pressure.
3. Once cooking is complete, use a natural release for 15 minutes; remove the lid carefully.
4. Ladle into individual serving bowls and eat warm. Bon appétit!

Italian-Style Asparagus Salad

Preparation Time: 10 minutes

Servings 4

Nutritional Values per serving: 230 Calories; 19.1g Fat; 10.1g Carbs; 7.9g Protein; 4.9g Sugars

Ingredients

- 1 pound asparagus, trimmed
- 2 tomatoes, diced
- 4 tablespoons olive oil
- 1 shallot, chopped
- 1 teaspoon garlic, minced
- Sea salt and ground black pepper, to taste
- 2 tablespoons lemon juice
- 1 tablespoon Dijon mustard
- 1/2 cup Romano cheese,grated
- 1 handful Italian parsley

Directions

1. Add 1 cup of water and metal trivet to the Instant Pot. Place asparagus on the trivet.
2. Secure the lid. Choose the "Manual" mode and cook for 1 minute under High pressure. Once cooking is complete, use a quick release; carefully remove the lid.
3. Toss the prepared asparagus with remaining ingredients; toss to combine well. Place in your refrigerator until ready to serve. Enjoy!

Pumpkin Porridge with Dried Cherries

Preparation Time: 25 minutes

Servings 4

Nutritional Values per serving: 201 Calories; 1.1g Fat; 51.8g Carbs; 5g Protein; 31.9g Sugars

Ingredients

- 2 ½ pounds pumpkin,cleaned and seeds removed
- 1/2 cup rolled oats
- 4 tablespoons honey
- 1/2 teaspoon ground cinnamon
- A pinch of salt
- A pinch of grated nutmeg
- 4 tablespoons dried berries
- 1 cup water

Directions

1. Add 1 ½ cups of water and a metal trivet to the Instant Pot. Now, place the pumpkin on the trivet.
2. Secure the lid. Choose the "Manual" mode and cook for 12 minutes under High pressure. Once cooking is complete, use a natural release; carefully remove the lid.
3. Then, purée the pumpkin in the food processor.
4. Wipe down the Instant Pot with a damp cloth. Add the remaining ingredients to the Instant Pot, including pumpkin purée.
5. Secure the lid. Choose the "Manual" mode and cook for 10 minutes under High pressure. Once cooking is complete, use a natural release; carefully remove the lid.

Easy Vegan Risotto

Preparation Time: 15 minutes

Servings 2

Nutritional Values per serving: 291 Calories; 20g Fat; 35.4g Carbs; 11.3g Protein; 2.8g Sugars

Ingredients

- 1 tablespoon olive oil
- 2 garlic cloves, minced
- 1 white onion, finely chopped
- 1 cup Arborio rice
- 1 cup water
- 1 cup vegetable stock
- 1/2 teaspoon dried basil
- 1/2 teaspoon dried oregano
- Sea salt and ground black pepper, to taste
- 1 teaspoon smoked paprika

Directions

1. Press the "Sauté" button to preheat your Instant Pot. Heat the oil and sauté the garlic and onion until tender and fragrant or about 3 minutes.
2. Add the remaining ingredients; stir to combine well.
3. Secure the lid. Choose the "Manual" mode and cook for 5 minutes under High pressure. Once cooking is complete, use a quick release; carefully remove the lid.
4. Ladle into individual bowls and serve warm. Enjoy!

Refreshing Bean Salad

Preparation Time: 35 minutes + chilling time

Servings 4

Nutritional Values per serving: 207 Calories; 5.1g Fat; 31.2g Carbs; 10.6g Protein; 2.3g Sugars

Ingredients

- 1 cup Great Northern beans
- 6 cups water
- 1 cucumber, peeled and sliced
- 1 red bell pepper, seeded and chopped
- 1 green bell pepper, seeded and chopped
- 1 teaspoon ground sumac
- 3 tablespoons extra-virgin olive oil
- 1 tablespoon fresh lime juice
- 1/4 cup fresh parsley leaves, roughly chopped
- 1/4 teaspoon freshly ground black pepper
- 1/2 teaspoon red pepper flakes
- Salt, to taste

Directions

1. Place beans and water in your Instant Pot.
2. Secure the lid. Choose the "Bean/Chili" mode and cook for 30 minutes under High pressure. Once cooking is complete, use a natural release; carefully remove the lid.
3. Allow the prepared beans to cool completely. Now, add the remaining ingredients to the Instant Pot.
4. Toss to combine and serve well chilled. Enjoy!

Root Vegetable and Noodle Soup

Preparation Time: 20 minutes

Servings 6

Nutritional Values per serving: 194 Calories; 5.4g Fat; 29.9g Carbs; 8g Protein; 5.1g Sugars

Ingredients

- 2 tablespoons olive oil
- 2 shallots, peeled and chopped
- 1 carrot, chopped
- 1 parsnip, chopped
- 1 turnip, chopped
- 3 garlic cloves, smashed
- 1 teaspoon cumin powder
- 1/2 teaspoon dried rosemary
- 1/2 teaspoon dried thyme
- 6 cups vegetable stock, preferably homemade
- 9 ounces vegan noodles
- 1 cup corn kernels
- Salt and freshly ground black pepper, to taste

Directions

1. Press the "Sauté" button to heat up your Instant Pot. Now, heat the oil and sauté the shallots with carrot, parsnip, and turnip until they have softened.
2. Stir in the garlic and cook an additional 40 seconds. Add cumin powder, rosemary, thyme, stock, and noodles.
3. Now, secure the lid and choose the "Soup" setting.
4. Cook for 7 minutes at High pressure. Once cooking is complete, use a quick release; remove the lid carefully.
5. Add corn kernels, cover with the lid, and cook in the residual heat for 5 to 6 minutes more. Season with salt and pepper.Taste adjust the seasoning and serve warm. Bon appétit!

Quinoa Pilaf with Cremini Mushrooms

Preparation Time: 15 minutes

Servings 4

Nutritional Values per serving: 401 Calories; 12.1g Fat; 60.2g Carbs; 14.1g Protein; 2.7g Sugars

Ingredients

- 2 cups dry quinoa
- 3 cups water
- 2 tablespoons olive oil
- 1 onion, chopped
- 1 bell pepper, chopped
- 2 garlic cloves, chopped
- 2 cups Cremini mushrooms, thinly sliced
- 1/2 teaspoon sea salt
- 1/3 teaspoon ground black pepper, or more to taste
- 1 teaspoon cayenne pepper
- 1/2 teaspoon dried dill
- 1/4 teaspoon ground bay leaf

Directions

1. Add quinoa and water to your Instant Pot.
2. Secure the lid. Choose the “Manual” mode and cook for 1 minute under High pressure. Once cooking is complete, use a natural release; carefully remove the lid.
3. Drain quinoa and set it aside.
4. Press the “Sauté” button to preheat your Instant Pot. Once hot, heat the oil.Then, sauté the onion until tender and translucent.
5. Add bell pepper, garlic, and mushrooms and continue to sauté for 1 to 2 minutes more or until they are fragrant. Stir the remaining ingredients into your Instant Pot.
6. Add the reserved quinoa and stir to combine well. Serve warm. Bon appétit!

Butternut Squash and Barley Bowl

Preparation Time: 45 minutes

Servings 4

Nutritional Values per serving: 360 Calories; 6.4g Fat; 70g Carbs; 8.7g Protein; 2.2g Sugars

Ingredients

- 2 tablespoons olive oil divided
- 2 cloves garlic, minced
- 1/2 cup scallions, chopped
- 2 cups butternut squash, peeled and cubed
- 1/2 teaspoon turmeric powder
- 2 cups barley, whole
- 4 ½ cups water
- Sea salt and ground black pepper, to taste

Directions

1. Press the "Sauté" button to preheat your Instant Pot. Once hot, heat the oil. Now, cook the garlic and scallions until tender.
2. Add the remaining ingredients and stir to combine.
3. Secure the lid. Choose the "Multigrain" mode and cook for 40 minutes under High pressure. Once cooking is complete, use a natural release; carefully remove the lid.
4. Ladle into individual bowls and serve warm.

Colorful Veggie and Coconut Soup

Preparation Time: 25 minutes

Servings 5

Nutritional Values per serving: 176 Calories; 13.1g Fat; 9.3g Carbs; 7.9g Protein; 3.4g Sugars

Ingredients

- 1 tablespoon olive oil
- 1/2 cup white onions, chopped
- 1 teaspoon garlic, minced
- 2 carrots, chopped
- 1 parsnip, chopped
- 1 celery, chopped
- 1 head cauliflower, cut into small florets
- 1 zucchini, diced
- 5 cups vegetable stock
- Sea salt and ground black pepper, to taste
- 1/2 cup coconut cream
- 2 tablespoons fresh cilantro, chopped

Directions

1. Press the "Sauté" button to preheat your Instant Pot. Now, heat the oil until sizzling.
2. Sauté the onion and garlic until tender. Add the carrots, parsnip, celery, cauliflower, zucchini, stock, salt, and black pepper, and stir to combine.
3. Secure the lid. Choose the "Soup" mode and cook for 20 minutes under High pressure. Once cooking is complete, use a quick release; carefully remove the lid.
4. Add coconut cream and seal the lid; let it sit until heated through. Ladle into soup bowls and serve garnished with fresh cilantro. Bon appétit!

Broccoli and Carrots with Peanut Sauce

Preparation Time: 10 minutes

Servings 4

Nutritional Values per serving: 90 Calories; 4.3g Fat; 9.3g Carbs; 5.2g Protein; 4.3g Sugars

Ingredients

- 1 ¼ cups water
- 1 pound broccoli florets
- 1 carrot, diced
- 1/2 teaspoon sea salt
- 1/2 teaspoon cayenne pepper
- 1/4 teaspoon ground white pepper
- For the Sauce:
- 4 tablespoons silky peanut butter
- 3 tablespoons water
- 1 tablespoon champagne vinegar
- 1 tablespoons poppy seeds

Directions

1. Add 1 ¼ cups of water to the base of your Instant Pot. Arrange broccoli and carrots in a steaming basket and transfer them to the Instant Pot.
2. Secure the lid, choose the "Manual" mode, and cook for 3 minutes at High pressure. Once cooking is complete, use a quick release; carefully remove the lid.
3. Season your vegetables with salt, cayenne pepper, and ground white pepper.
4. Meanwhile, in a mixing bowl, thoroughly combine peanut butter, water, vinegar, and poppy seeds.
5. Serve steamed broccoli and carrots with the peanut sauce on the side.Bon appétit!

Delicious Old-Fashioned Chili

Preparation Time: 15 minutes

Servings 6

Nutritional Values per serving: 204 Calories; 6.5g Fat; 27.9g Carbs; 10.4g Protein; 6.9g Sugars

Ingredients

- 2 tablespoons olive oil
- 1 red onion, chopped
- 3 cloves garlic minced or pressed
- 1 red bell pepper, diced
- 1 green bell pepper, diced
- 1 red chili pepper, minced
- Sea salt and ground black pepper, to taste
- 1 teaspoon cayenne pepper
- 1/2 teaspoon ground cumin
- 2 cups vegetable stock
- 2 ripe tomatoes, chopped
- 2 (15-ounce cans beans, drained and rinsed
- 1 handful fresh cilantro leaves, chopped
- 1/2 cup tortilla chips

Directions

1. Press the "Sauté" button to preheat your Instant Pot. Now, heat the oil until sizzling.
2. Sauté the onion tender and translucent. Add garlic, peppers, salt, and pepper; continue to sauté until they are tender.
3. Now, stir in cayenne pepper, cumin, stock, tomatoes, and beans.
4. Secure the lid. Choose the "Manual" mode and cook for 10 minutes under High pressure. Once cooking is complete, use a quick release; carefully remove the lid.
5. Divide chili between six serving bowls; top with fresh cilantro and tortilla chips. Enjoy!

Traditional Russian Borscht

Preparation Time: 15 minutes

Servings 4

Nutritional Values per serving: 183 Calories; 7.3g Fat; 22.5g Carbs; 8.4g Protein; 7.7g Sugars

Ingredients

- 1 ½ tablespoons olive oil
- 1/2 cup onions, chopped
- 2 garlic cloves, pressed
- Kosher salt and ground black pepper, to taste
- 1/2 pound potatoes, peeled and diced
- 2 carrots, chopped
- 1/2 pound beets, peeled and coarsely shredded
- 2 tablespoons red-wine vinegar
- 1 tomato, chopped
- 4 cups vegetable stock
- 1/2 teaspoon caraway seeds
- 1/4 cup fresh dill, roughly chopped

Directions

1. Press the “Sauté” button to preheat your Instant Pot. Heat the oil and cook the onions and garlic until tender and fragrant.
2. Add the remaining ingredients, except for fresh dill.
3. Secure the lid. Choose the “Manual” mode and cook for 10 minutes under High pressure. Once cooking is complete, use a natural release; carefully remove the lid.
4. Serve the soup with chopped fresh dill. Enjoy!

Winter Curry Cabbage

Preparation Time: 20 minutes

Servings 4

Nutritional Values per serving: 223 Calories; 8.2g Fat; 33.8g Carbs; 7.6g Protein; 15.1g Sugars

Ingredients

- 2 tablespoons olive oil
- 1 medium-sized leek, chopped
- 2 cloves garlic, smashed
- 1 ½ pounds white cabbage, shredded
- 1 cup vegetable broth
- 1 cup tomatoes, puréed
- 1 parsnip, chopped
- 2 carrots, chopped
- 2 stalks celery, chopped
- 1 turnip, chopped
- 1/2 tablespoon fresh lime juice
- 1 teaspoon dried basil
- 1/2 teaspoon dried dill
- 1 teaspoon ground coriander
- 1 teaspoon ground turmeric
- 1 bay leaf
- Kosher salt and ground black pepper, to taste

- 1 (14-ounce can coconut milk

Directions

1. Press the "Sauté" button to preheat your Instant Pot. Now, heat the oil and cook the leeks and garlic until tender and fragrant.
2. After that, add the remaining ingredients; stir to combine well.
3. Secure the lid. Choose the "Manual" mode and cook for 12 minutes under High pressure. Once cooking is complete, use a natural release; carefully remove the lid.
4. Ladle into soup bowls and serve immediately.

The Easiest Hummus Ever

Preparation Time: 35 minutes

Servings 8

Nutritional Values per serving: 186 Calories; 7.7g Fat; 22.8g Carbs; 7.6g Protein; 4g Sugars

Ingredients

- 10 cups water
- 3/4 pound dried chickpeas, soaked
- 2 tablespoons tahini
- 1/2 lemon, juiced
- 1 teaspoon granulated garlic
- Salt and black pepper, to taste
- 1/3 teaspoon ground cumin
- 1/2 teaspoon cayenne pepper
- 1/2 teaspoon dried basil
- 3 tablespoon olive oil

Directions

1. Add water and chickpeas to the Instant Pot. Secure the lid.
2. Choose the "Manual" mode and cook for 25 minutes under High pressure.Once cooking is complete, use a natural release; carefully remove the lid.
3. Now, drain your chickpeas, reserving the liquid. Transfer chickpeas to a food processor. Add tahini, lemon juice, and seasonings.
4. Puree until it is creamy; gradually pour in the reserved liquid and olive oil until the mixture is smooth and uniform. Serve with a few sprinkles of cayenne pepper. Bon appétit!

Green Beans with Shiitake Mushrooms

Preparation Time: 25 minutes

Servings 4

Nutritional Values per serving: 119 Calories; 7.6g Fat; 12.6g Carbs; 2.6g Protein; 2.6g Sugars

Ingredients

- 2 cups water
- 6 dried shiitake mushrooms
- 2 tablespoons sesame oil
- 2 cloves garlic, minced
- 1/2 cup scallions, chopped
- 1 ½ pounds green beans,fresh or frozen (and thawed
- 1/4 teaspoon ground black pepper
- 1/2 teaspoon red pepper flakes, crushed
- 1 bay leaf
- Sea salt, to taste

Directions

1. Press the "Sauté" button and bring the water to a rapid boil; remove from the heat; add the dried shiitake mushrooms.
2. Allow the mushrooms to sit for 15 minutes to rehydrate. Then cut the mushrooms into slices; reserve the mushroom stock.
3. Wipe down the Instant Pot with a kitchen cloth. Press the "Sauté" button to preheat your Instant Pot. Once hot, heat the sesame oil.
4. Then, sauté the garlic and scallions until tender and aromatic. Add green beans, black pepper, red pepper, bay leaf, salt, reserved mushrooms and stock; stir to combine well.
5. Secure the lid. Choose the "Manual" mode and cook for 4 minutes under High pressure. Once cooking is complete, use a quick release; carefully remove the lid. Serve warm.

Lentil Chipotle Curry

Preparation Time:: 20 minutes

Servings: 3

Ingredients:

- 1 cup brown lentils; rinsed and picked over
- 1/2 medium onion; chopped.
- 1/2 medium green bell pepper; chopped.
- 1/2 tbsp. canola oil
- 1 chipotle in adobo sauce; seeded and chopped.
- 1/4 cup sun-dried tomatoes; chopped.
- 1/2 tsp. ground cumin
- 1 garlic clove; chopped.
- 1½ tbsp. chili powder
- 1 can (1/4 oz. diced tomatoes
- 2 cups vegetable broth
- Salt; to taste

Directions:

1. Add oil with onion and bell pepper to Instant Pot and select *Sauté* to cook for 2 minutes
2. Stir in garlic and chili powder; then sauté for 1 minute.
3. Add all the remaining Ingredientsand secure the lid
4. Cook on the *Manual* function for 12 minutes on high pressure.
5. When it beeps; do a Natural release for 10 minutes; then release the remaining steam with a Quick release,
6. Garnish with chopped cilantro and shredded Cheddar cheese, Serve.

Chorizo Pinto Beans

Preparation Time:: 52 minutes

Servings: 3

Ingredients:

- 1 cup dry pinto beans
- 1/2 tbsp. cooking oil
- 2 oz. dry (Spanish chorizo
- 1/2 yellow onion
- 1½ garlic cloves
- 1 bay leaf
- 1/2 tsp. freshly cracked pepper
- 1½ cups chicken broth
- 7½ oz. can diced tomatoes

Directions:

1. Add oil, chorizo, garlic and onion to Instant Pot. *Sauté* for 5 minutes.
2. Stir in beans, pepper and bay leaf. Cook for 1 minute then add the broth
3. Cover and secure the lid. Turn its pressure release handle to the sealing position.
4. Cook on the *Manual* function with high pressure for 35 minutes
5. When it beeps; do a Natural release for 20 minutes.
6. Stir in diced tomatoes and cook for 7 minutes on the *Sauté* setting. Serve hot with boiled white rice or tortilla chips.

White Beans Curry

- Preparation Time:: 35 minutes
- Servings: 6

Ingredients:

- 1 lb. white beans; soaked and rinsed
- 1/2 tsp. red pepper
- 1/2 tsp. ground turmeric
- 1 - 2 tsp. salt
- 1 bay leaf
- 6 cups unsalted vegetable broth
- 1 tbsp. onion powder
- 2 tsp. garlic powder

Directions:

1. Add all the Ingredientsto Instant Pot
2. Cover and secure the lid. Turn its pressure release handle to the sealing position.
3. Cook on the *Bean/Chili* function on the default settings.
4. When it beeps; do a Natural release for 20 minutes, Stir and serve hot with boiled white rice

Chicken and Brown Rice

Preparation Time:: 43 minutes

Servings: 6

Ingredients:

- 2 lb. chicken thigh; boneless, skinless
- 2 cups brown rice; raw
- 1 medium onion
- 3 garlic cloves
- 2 cups baby carrots
- 2 cups cremini mushrooms
- 1 tbsp. olive oil
- 2¼ cups chicken broth
- 1/8 tsp. salt
- 1/8 tsp. ground black pepper
- 10 oz. soup; cream of chicken, canned, condensed
- 2 tbsp. Worcestershire sauce
- 1 tbsp. fresh thyme

Directions:

1. Add oil, garlic, vegetables and onions to Instant Pot. *Sauté* for 2 minutes
2. Add all the remaining Ingredientsto the cooker. Place the chicken pieces on top.

3. Cover and secure the lid. Turn its pressure release handle to the sealing position.
4. Cook on the *Manual* function with high pressure for 31 minutes
5. When it beeps; do a Natural release for 7 minutes
6. Remove the chicken and shred its meat. Add the meat back to the rice, Stir and serve warm.

Veg Rice

Preparation Time:: 27 minutes

Servings: 3

Ingredients:

- 1 cup basmati rice; rinsed
- 3 tbsp. olive oil
- 1/2 large onion; diced small
- 1/2 cup green bell pepper; chopped.
- 1/2 cup carrots; chopped.
- 1/2 cup green onion; chopped.
- 1 large garlic clove; finely diced
- 1/2 cup frozen garden peas
- 3/4 cup vegetable stock
- Salt; to taste
- Black pepper; to taste

Directions:

1. Add oil and all the vegetables to Instant Pot and *Sauté* for 7 minutes
2. Stir in all the remaining Ingredientsexcept the butter.
3. Cover and secure the lid. Turn its pressure release handle to the sealing position.
4. Cook on the *Manual* function with high pressure for 5 minutes
5. When it beeps; do a Natural release for 7 minutes, Stir and serve warm.

Mung Bean Curry

Preparation Time:: 35 minutes

Servings: 4

Ingredients:

- 1/2 cup raw mung beans
- 1/2 cup chopped onions
- 1½ tbsp. cooking oil
- 1 bay leaf
- 1 cup vegetable broth
- 1/4 tsp. turmeric
- 1/2 tsp. coriander powder
- 1 tsp. chili powder
- 1/2 tbsp. grated garlic
- 1/4 tbsp. grated ginger
- 3/4 cup water
- 1 cup chopped baby spinach
- Salt; to taste

Directions:

1. Add oil and onions to Instant Pot. *Sauté* for 5 minutes
2. Stir ginger, garlic paste and bay leaf. Cook for 1 minute then add all the spices
3. Add mung beans, broth and water to the pot.

4. Cover and secure the lid. Turn its pressure release handle to the sealing position.
5. Cook on the *Manual* function with high pressure for 15 minutes
6. When it beeps; do a Natural release for 20 minutes
7. Stir in spinach and cook for 3 minutes on the *Sauté* setting. Serve hot with boiled white rice,

Mexican Rice

Preparation Time:: 21 minutes

Servings: 3

Ingredients:

- 1 cup long-grain white rice
- 1 tbsp. avocado oil
- 1/4 cup onion; chopped.
- 2 garlic cloves; finely chopped.
- 1/2 tsp. salt
- 2 tbsp. crushed tomatoes
- 2 tbsp. cilantro; chopped.
- 2 tbsp. sun-dried tomatoes
- 2 cups chicken stock
- 1/4 tsp. cumin
- 1/4 tsp. garlic powder
- 1/4 tsp. smoked paprika

Directions:

1. Add oil, onion and garlic to Instant Pot. *Sauté* for 3 minutes.
2. Stir in rice and mix well with the onion.
3. Add all the remaining Ingredientsto the cooker.
4. Cover and secure the lid. Turn its pressure release handle to the sealing position
5. Cook on the *Manual* function with high pressure for 8 minutes.
6. When it beeps; do a Natural release, Stir and serve warm.

Pea & Corn Rice

Preparation Time:: 13 minutes

Servings: 3

Ingredients:

- 1/2 cup frozen garden peas
- 1 cup basmati rice; rinsed
- 1½ tbsp. olive oil
- 1/2 large onion; diced small
- Salt; to taste
- 1½ tbsp. chopped cilantro stalks
- 1 large garlic clove; finely diced
- 1/2 tsp. turmeric powder
- 1/2 cup frozen sweet corn kernels
- 3/4 cup chicken stock
- 1 dollop of butter

Directions:

1. Add oil and onions to Instant Pot and *Sauté* for 5 minutes
2. Stir in all the remaining Ingredientsexcept the butter
3. Cover and secure the lid. Turn its pressure release handle to the sealing position.
4. Cook on the *Manual* function with high pressure for 3 minutes
5. When it beeps; do a Natural release for 7 minutes.
6. Stir in butter and let it melt into the rice, Serve warm.

Lentil Risotto

Preparation Time:: 30 minutes

Servings: 2

Ingredients:

- 1/2 cup dry lentils; soaked overnight
- 1 garlic clove; lightly mashed
- 2 cups vegetable stock
- 1/2 tbsp. olive oil
- 1/2 medium onion; chopped.
- 1/2 celery stalk; chopped.
- 1 sprig parsley; chopped.
- 1/2 cup Arborio (short-grain Italian rice

Directions:

1. Add oil and onions to Instant Pot and *Sauté* for 5 minutes.
2. Add all the remaining ingredient to Instant Pot.
3. Cover and secure the lid. Turn its pressure release handle to the sealing position
4. Cook on the *Manual* function with high pressure for 15 minutes
5. When it beeps; do a Natural release for 20 minutes, Stir and serve hot with boiled white rice

Cilantro Rice

Preparation Time:: 21 minutes

Servings: 6

Ingredients:

- 1⅓ cup white rice
- 1/2 tbsp. butter
- 1/2 yellow onion; diced
- 1 garlic clove; minced
- 2 cups water
- 1/2 tbsp. chicken bouillon
- 1/2 cup peas
- 1/2 tsp. cumin
- 2 oz. can green chilies
- 1/4 bunch cilantro; chopped.
- 3/4 tsp. fresh lime juice
- Salt; to taste

Directions:

1. Add oil, onion and garlic to Instant Pot and *Sauté* for 4 minutes.
2. Add all the remaining Ingredientsto the cooker
3. Cover and secure the lid. Turn its pressure release handle to the sealing position
4. Cook on the *Manual* function with high pressure for 7 minutes.
5. When it beeps; do a Natural release and open the instant pot lid. Garnish with fresh cilantro and serve.

Almond Risotto

Preparation Time:: 15 minutes

Servings: 3

Ingredients:

- 1/2 cup Arborio (short-grain Italian rice
- 2 cups vanilla almond milk
- 2 tbsp. agave syrup
- 1 tsp. vanilla extract
- 1/4 cup toasted almond flakes

Directions:

1. Add all the Ingredientsto Instant Pot.
2. Cover and secure the lid. Turn its pressure release handle to the sealing position
3. Cook on the *Manual* function with high pressure for 5 minutes
4. When it beeps; do a Natural release for 20 minutes, Garnish with almond flakes and serve.

Black Bean Burrito

Preparation Time:: 22 minutes

Servings: 4

Ingredients:

- 1/2 tbsp. olive oil
- 1/2 small onion; diced
- 1/2 can black beans; rinsed
- 1/2 cup long-grain white rice; uncooked
- 1/2 cup salsa
- 1 cup chicken broth
- 1/2 garlic clove; minced
- 1/2 tsp. chili powder
- 1/4 tsp. Kosher salt
- 3/4 lb. boneless; skinless chicken thighs, cut into 1-inch pieces
- 2 tbsp. chopped cilantro
- 2 tbsp. Cheddar cheese

Directions:

1. Add oil with onion and garlic to Instant Pot and select *Sauté* to cook for 2 minutes.
2. Add all the remaining Ingredientsand secure the lid.
3. Cook on the *Manual* function for 10 minutes on high pressure
4. When it beeps; do a Natural release for 10 minutes; then release the remaining steam with a Quick release
5. Garnish with chopped cilantro and shredded Cheddar. Serve.

Red Bean Curry

Preparation Time:: 34 minutes

Servings: 4

Ingredients:

- 1/2 cup raw red beans
- 1½ tbsp. cooking oil
- 1/2 cup chopped onions
- 1 bay leaf
- 1/2 tbsp. grated garlic
- 1/4 tbsp. grated ginger
- 3/4 cup water
- 1 cup fresh tomato puree
- 1/2 green chili; finely chopped.
- 1/4 tsp. turmeric
- 1/2 tsp. coriander powder
- 1 tsp. chili powder
- 1 cup chopped baby spinach
- Salt; to taste
- 1/2 cup fresh cilantro

Directions:

1. Add oil and onions to Instant Pot. *Sauté* for 5 minutes
2. Stir ginger, garlic paste, green chili and bay leaf. Cook for 1 minute then add all the spices
3. Add red beans, tomato puree and water to the pot.
4. Cover and secure the lid. Turn its pressure release handle to the sealing position.
5. Cook on the *Manual* function with high pressure for 15 minutes
6. When it beeps; do a Natural release for 20 minutes
7. Stir in spinach and cook for 3 minutes on the *Sauté* setting. Serve hot with boiled white rice

Chickpea Rice

Preparation Time:: 48 minutes

Servings: 8

Ingredients:

- 4½ cups brown rice; rinsed and drained
- 1/2 cup chickpeas; soaked
- 8 bacon strips; chopped.
- 4 tbsp. cooking oil
- 2 onions; minced
- 6 cups vegetable broth
- 1/2 cup chopped cilantro

Directions:

1. Add oil and onion to Instant Pot. *Sauté* for 3 minutes
2. Stir in bacon. Sauté for 5 minutes
3. Add all the remaining Ingredientsto the cooker.
4. Cover and secure the lid. Turn its pressure release handle to the sealing position.
5. Cook on the *Manual* function with high pressure for 30 minutes
6. When it beeps; do a Natural release and open the instant pot lid. Stir and serve warm.

Fennel Risotto

Preparation Time:: 29 minutes

Servings: 3

Ingredients:

- 1/4 medium fennel; diced
- 1/2 medium brown onion; finely diced
- 1 tbsp. olive oil
- 1/4 bunch of asparagus; diced
- 1/4 tsp. salt
- 1 garlic clove; chopped.
- 1 cup Arborio risotto rice
- 1 cup vegetable stock
- 1 cup chicken stock
- 1 tbsp. butter
- 3 tbsp. white wine
- Zest of 1/4 lemon
- 1/4 cup grated Parmesan cheese

Directions:

1. Add oil, onion, fennel and asparagus to Instant Pot and *Sauté* for 4 minutes.
2. Add all the remaining Ingredients(except the cheese to the cooker.
3. Cover and secure the lid. Turn its pressure release handle to the sealing position
4. Cook on the *Manual* function with high pressure for 10 minutes.
5. When it beeps; do a Natural release and open the instant pot lid. Stir in cheese and serve.

Black Bean Gravy

Preparation Time:: 35 minutes

Servings: 6

Ingredients:

- 1 lb. black beans; sorted and rinsed
- 1/2 tsp. red pepper
- 1/2 tsp. ground turmeric
- 6 cups unsalted vegetable broth
- 1 tbsp. onion powder
- 2 tsp. garlic powder
- 1 tsp. salt
- 1 bay leaf

Directions:

1. Add all the Ingredientsto Instant Pot.
2. Cover and secure the lid. Turn its pressure release handle to the sealing position
3. Cook on the *Beans/Chili* function on the default settings.
4. When it beeps; do a Natural release for 20 minutes, Stir and serve hot with boiled white rice

Mushrooms Risotto

Preparation Time:: 30 minutes

Servings: 2

Ingredients:

- 1/2 cup cremini mushrooms; sliced
- 1/2 cup Arborio (short-grain Italian rice
- 1/2 tbsp. olive oil
- 1/2 medium onion; chopped.
- 1 garlic clove; lightly mashed
- 2 cups vegetable stock
- 1/2 celery stalk; chopped.
- 1 sprig parsley; chopped.

Directions:

1. Add oil and onions to Instant Pot and *Sauté* for 5 minutes
2. Add all the remaining Ingredientsto Instant Pot.
3. Cover and secure the lid. Turn its pressure release handle to the sealing position
4. Cook on the *Manual* function with high pressure for 15 minutes
5. When it beeps; do a Natural release for 20 minutes, Stir and serve hot with boiled white rice.

Lentils Spinach Stew

Preparation Time:: 34 minutes

Servings: 4

Ingredients:

- 1 cup chopped baby spinach
- 1/2 cup raw lentils
- 1½ tbsp. cooking oil
- 1/2 cup chopped onions
- 1 bay leaf
- 1/2 tbsp. grated garlic
- 1/4 tbsp. grated ginger
- 3/4 cup water
- 1 cup fresh tomato puree
- 1/2 green chili; finely chopped.
- 1/4 tsp. turmeric
- 1/2 tsp. coriander powder
- 1 tsp. chili powder
- Salt; to taste
- 1/2 cup fresh cilantro

Directions:

1. Add oil and onions to Instant Pot. *Sauté* for 5 minutes.
2. Stir ginger, garlic paste and bay leaf. Cook for 1 minute then add all the spices
3. Add lentils, tomato puree and water to the pot
4. Cover and secure the lid. Turn its pressure release handle to the sealing position.
5. Cook on the *Manual* function with high pressure for 15 minutes.
6. When it beeps; do a Natural release for 20 minutes
7. Stir in spinach and cook for 3 minutes on the *Sauté* setting. Serve hot with boiled white rice

Chorizo Red Beans

Preparation Time:: 52 minutes

Servings: 3

Ingredients:

- 1 cup red beans; soaked and rinsed
- Freshly cracked pepper
- 1/2 tbsp. cooking oil
- 2 oz. dry (Spanish chorizo
- 1/2 yellow onion
- 1½ garlic cloves
- 1 bay leaf
- 1½ cups reduced sodium chicken broth
- 7½ oz. can diced tomatoes

Directions:

1. Add oil, chorizo, garlic and onion to Instant Pot. *Sauté* for 5 minutes.
2. Stir in beans, pepper and bay leaf. Cook for 1 minute; then add the broth
3. Cover and secure the lid. Turn its pressure release handle to the sealing position.
4. Cook on the *Manual* function with high pressure for 35 minutes
5. When it beeps; do a Natural release for 20 minutes.
6. Stir in diced tomatoes and cook for 7 minutes on the *Sauté* setting. Serve hot with boiled white rice or tortilla chips.

Coconut Risotto

Preparation Time:: 15 minutes

Servings: 3

Ingredients:

- 1/2 cup Arborio (short-grain Italian rice
- 2 cups coconut milk
- 2 tbsp. coconut sugar
- 1/4 cup toasted coconut flakes
- 1 tsp. vanilla extract

Directions:

1. Add all the Ingredientsto Instant Pot. Cover and secure the lid. Turn its pressure release handle to the sealing position.
2. Cook on the *Manual* function with high pressure for 5 minutes
3. When it beeps; do a Natural release for 20 minutes, Garnish with coconut flakes and serve.

Potato Rice

Preparation Time:: 15 minutes

Servings: 3

Ingredients:

- 3 medium-sized potatoes; diced
- 1 cup basmati rice; rinsed
- 1½ tbsp. olive oil
- 1/2 large onion; diced small
- 1½ tbsp. chopped cilantro stalks
- 1 large garlic clove; finely diced
- 1/2 tsp. turmeric powder
- 1 cup chicken stock
- 1 tsp. butter
- Salt; to taste

Directions:

1. Add oil and all the vegetables to Instant Pot and *Sauté* for 5 minutes.
2. Stir in all the remaining Ingredientsexcept the butter.
3. Cover and secure the lid. Turn its pressure release handle to the sealing position.
4. Cook on the *Manual* function with high pressure for 5 minutes.
5. When it beeps; do a Natural release for 7 minutes
6. Stir in butter and let it melt into the rice, Serve warm.

Bean Mustard Curry

Serving: 4

Preparation Time: 10 minutes

Cooking Time: 14 minutes

Ingredients

- ½ cup ketchup
- ½ tablespoon olive oil
- 2 tablespoons molasses
- 2 teaspoons mustard powder
- ¼ teaspoon ground black pepper
- 1 ½ slices bacon, chopped
- ½ medium onion, chopped
- ½ small green bell pepper, chopped
- 1 ½ cans navy beans, rinsed and drained
- 1 teaspoon apple cider vinegar
- 2 tablespoons chopped cilantro (garnish

Directions

1. Select the "Sauté" function on your Instant Pot and add the oil with onion, bacon and bell pepper. Cook for 6 minutes.
2. Add all the remaining ingredients and secure the lid.
3. Cook on the "Manual" function for 8 minutes on high pressure.
4. After the beep, do a Natural release for 10 minutes, then release the remaining steam with a Quick release.
5. Garnish with chopped cilantro on top.
6. Serve.

Nutrition Values Per Serving:

Calories: 373

Carbohydrate:64.5g

Protein: 21.2g

Fat: 4.7g

Sugar: 16.1g

Sodium: 507mg

White Bean Curry

Serving: 4

Preparation Time: 5 minutes

Cookingtime: 30 minutes

Ingredients

- 1 lb. white beans, soaked and rinsed
- ½ teaspoon red pepper
- ½ teaspoon ground turmeric
- 1 tablespoon onion powder
- 2 teaspoons garlic powder
- 1-2 teaspoons salt
- 1 bay leaf
- 6 cups unsalted vegetable broth
- Boiled white rice to serve

Directions

1. Add all the listed ingredients except the white rice to the Instant Pot.
2. Cover and secure the lid. Turn its pressure release handle to the sealing position.
3. Cook on the "Bean/Chilli" function on the default settings.
4. After the beep, do a Natural release for 20 minutes.
5. Stir and serve hot with boiled white rice.

Nutrition Values Per Serving:

Calories:286

Carbohydrate: 54.1g

Protein: 19.1g

Fat: 1.2g

Sugar: 5.2g

Sodium: 612mg

Pea & Corn Rice

Serving: 3

Preparation Time: 5 minutes

Cooking Time: 8 minutes

Ingredients

- 1 cup basmati rice, rinsed
- 1 ½ tablespoons olive oil
- ½ large onion, diced small
- Salt, to taste
- 1 ½ tablespoons chopped cilantro stalks
- 1 large garlic clove, finely diced
- ½ teaspoon turmeric powder
- ½ cup frozen sweet corn kernels
- ½ cup frozen garden peas
- ¾ cup chicken stock
- 1 dollop of butter

Directions

1. Add the oil and onions to the Instant Pot and "Sauté" for 5 minutes.
2. Stir in all the remaining ingredients except the butter.
3. Cover and secure the lid. Turn its pressure release handle to the sealing position.

4. Cook on the "Manual" function with high pressure for 3 minutes.
5. After the beep, do a Natural release for 7 minutes.
6. Stir in butter and let it melt into the rice.
7. Serve warm.

Nutrition Values Per Serving:

Calories: 356

Carbohydrate: 61.3g

Protein: 7.1g

Fat: 9.2g

Sugar: 3.6g

Sodium: 363mg

Shrimp & Rice Paella

Serving: 8

Preparation Time: 10 minutes

Cooking Time: 10 minutes

Ingredients

- 32 oz. frozen wild-caught shrimp
- 16 oz. jasmine rice
- 4 oz. butter
- 4 oz. chopped fresh parsley
- 2 teaspoons sea salt
- ½ teaspoon black pepper
- 2 pinches crushed red pepper
- 2 medium lemons, juiced
- 2 pinches saffron
- 24 oz. chicken broth
- 8 garlic cloves, minced

Directions

1. Add all the ingredients to the Instant Pot.
2. Place the shrimp on top.
3. Cover and secure the lid. Turn its pressure release handle to the sealing position.
4. Cook on the “Manual” function with high pressure for 10 minutes.

5. After the beep, do a Natural release for 7 minutes.
6. If needed, remove the shells of the shrimp and then add the shrimp back to the rice.
7. Stir and serve warm.

Nutrition Values Per Serving:

Calories: 437

Carbohydrate: 49.1g

Protein: 30.6g

Fat: 13.7g

Sugar: 0.8g

Sodium: 1086mg

Black Beans with Chorizo

Serving: 3

Preparation Time: 5 minutes

Cookingtime: 47 minutes

Ingredients

- ½ tablespoon cooking oil
- 2 oz. dry (Spanish chorizo
- ½ yellow onion
- 1 ½ garlic cloves
- 1 cup black beans, soaked and rinsed
- 1 bay leaf
- ½ teaspoon cracked pepper
- 1 ½ cups sodium-reduced chicken broth
- 1 cup (7.1 oz. tomatoes, diced
- Boiled white rice or tortilla chips to serve

Directions

1. Add the oil, chorizo, garlic and onion to the Instant Pot. "Sauté" for 5 minutes.
2. Stir in beans, pepper and bay leaf. Cook for 1 minute, then add the chicken broth.
3. Cover and secure the lid. Turn its pressure release handle to the sealing position.

4. Cook on the "Manual" function with high pressure for 35 minutes.
5. After the beep, do a Natural release for 15-20 minutes.
6. Stir in diced tomatoes and cook for 7 minutes on the "Sauté" setting.
7. Serve hot with boiled white rice or tortilla chips.

Nutrition Values Per Serving:

Calories: 324

Carbohydrate: 48.8g

Protein: 21.3g

Fat: 5.6g

Sugar: 5.3g

Sodium: 647mg

Brown Chicken Rice

Serving: 6

Preparation Time: 10 minutes

Cooking Time: 33 minutes

Ingredients

- 1 medium onion
- 3 garlic cloves
- 2 cups baby carrots
- 2 cups cremini mushrooms
- 2 cups brown rice, raw
- 1 tablespoon olive oil
- 2 ¼ cups chicken broth
- 2 lbs. chicken thigh, boneless, skinless
- ⅛ teaspoon salt
- ⅛ teaspoon ground black pepper
- 10 oz. soup, cream of chicken, canned, condensed
- 2 tablespoons Worcestershire sauce
- 1 tablespoon fresh thyme

Directions

1. Add the oil, garlic, vegetables and onions to the Instant Pot. "Sauté" for 2 minutes.
2. Add all the remaining ingredients to the cooker. Place the chicken pieces on top.

3. Cover and secure the lid. Turn its pressure release handle to the sealing position.
4. Cook on the "Manual" function with high pressure for 31 minutes.
5. After the beep, do a Natural release for 7 minutes.
6. Remove the chicken and shred its meat. Add the meat back to the rice.
7. Stir and serve warm.

Nutrition Values Per Serving:

Calories: 606

Carbohydrate: 58.8g

Protein: 52.4g

Fat: 16.6g

Sugar: 4.7g

Sodium: 897mg

Mushroom Risotto

Serving: 2

Preparation Time: 10 minutes

Cooking Time: 20 minutes

Ingredients

- ½ cup cremini mushrooms, sliced
- ½ tablespoon olive oil
- ½ medium onion, chopped
- ½ celery stalk, chopped
- 1 sprig parsley, chopped
- ½ cup Arborio (short-grain Italian rice
- 1 garlic clove, lightly mashed
- 2 cups vegetable stock

Directions

1. Add the oil and onions to the Instant Pot and "Sauté" for 5 minutes.
2. Add all the remaining ingredients to the Instant Pot.
3. Cover and secure the lid. Turn its pressure release handle to the sealing position.
4. Cook on the "Manual" function with high pressure for 15 minutes.
5. After the beep, do a Natural release for 20 minutes.
6. Stir and serve hot.

Nutrition Values Per Serving:

Calories: 226

Carbohydrate: 42.7g

Protein: 4.4g

Fat: 3.9g

Sugar: 2.3g

Sodium: 59mg

Mexican-Style Rice

Serving: 3

Preparation Time: 10 minutes

Cooking Time: 11 minutes

Ingredients

- 1 tablespoon avocado oil
- ¼ cup onion, chopped
- 2 garlic cloves, finely chopped
- 1 cup long-grain white rice
- ½ teaspoon salt
- 2 tablespoons crushed tomatoes
- 2 cups chicken stock
- ¼ teaspoon cumin
- ¼ teaspoon garlic powder
- ¼ teaspoon smoked paprika
- 2 tablespoons cilantro, chopped
- 2 tablespoons sun-dried tomatoes

Directions

1. Add the oil, onion and garlic to the Instant Pot. "Sauté" for 3 minutes.
2. Stir in rice and mix well with the onions.
3. Add all the remaining ingredients to the cooker.

4. Cover and secure the lid. Turn its pressure release handle to the sealing position.
5. Cook on the "Manual" function with high pressure for 8 minutes.
6. After the beep, do a Natural release.
7. Stir and serve warm.

Nutrition Values Per Serving:

Calories: 252

Carbohydrate: 53.1g

Protein: 5.6g

Fat: 1.5g

Sugar: 1.9g

Sodium: 922mg

Beef Rice

Serving: 3

Preparation Time: 5 minutes

Cooking Time: 16 minutes

Ingredients

- ½ tablespoon olive oil
- ½ lb. lean ground beef
- ½ cup diced red onion
- ½ teaspoon chili powder
- ¼ teaspoon ground cumin
- ¼ teaspoon salt
- ½ cup long-grain white rice, rinsed well and drained
- 1 cup water
- 1 cup chunky salsa
- 1 cup black beans, rinsed and drained
- ½ cup cooked corn kernels
- 1 tablespoon chopped fresh cilantro to garnish (optional

Directions

1. Add the oil and onion to the Instant Pot. "Sauté" for 3 minutes.
2. Stir in beef, cumin, salt and chili powder. Sauté for 5 minutes.

3. Add all the remaining ingredients to the cooker.
4. Cover and secure the lid. Turn its pressure release handle to the sealing position.
5. Cook on the "Manual" function with high pressure for 8 minutes.
6. After the beep, do a Natural release and remove the lid.
7. Stir and serve warm.

Nutrition Values Per Serving:

Calories: 378

Carbohydrate: 43.5g

Protein: 31.6g

Fat: 8.8g

Sugar: 5g

Sodium: 868mg

Cauliflower Risotto

Serving: 8

Preparation Time: 10 minutes

Cooking Time: 33 minutes

Ingredients

- 2 small heads of cauliflower, cut in chunks
- 6 tablespoons olive oil, divided
- Salt and freshly ground black pepper, to taste
- 1 cup freshly grated Parmesan cheese, divided
- 2 tablespoons olive oil
- 2 large onions, diced
- 4 garlic cloves, minced
- 2 cups pearl barley
- 6 cups vegetable or chicken broth
- 4 sprigs thyme
- 2 tablespoons butter
- 4 tablespoons chopped fresh parsley to garnish (optional

Directions

1. Add the oil, garlic and onion to the Instant Pot. “Sauté” for 3 minutes.
2. Stir in cauliflower chunks and “Sauté” for 5 minutes.

3. Add all the remaining ingredients to the cooker, except the cheese and butter.
4. Cover and secure the lid. Turn its pressure release handle to the sealing position.
5. Cook on the "Manual" function with high pressure for 25 minutes.
6. After the beep, do a Natural release and remove the lid.
7. Stir in butter and cheese.
8. Serve warm.

Nutrition Values Per Serving:

Calories: 372

Carbohydrate: 48.2g

Protein: 8.4g

Fat: 18.8g

Sugar: 1g

Sodium: 69mg

Vegetable & Corn Rice

Serving: 3

Preparation Time: 5 minutes

Cooking Time: 12 minutes

Ingredients

- 1 cup basmati rice, rinsed
- 1 ½ tablespoons olive oil
- ½ large onion, diced small
- Salt, to taste
- 1 ½ tablespoons chopped cilantro stalks
- 1 large garlic clove, finely diced
- ½ heaped teaspoon turmeric powder
- ½ cup frozen sweet corn kernels
- ½ cup carrots, chopped
- ¼ cup green onions, chopped
- ¼ cup bell peppers, chopped
- ½ cup frozen garden peas
- 1 cup chicken stock
- Dollop of butter, to finish

Directions

1. Add the oil and all the vegetables to the Instant Pot and "Sauté" for 5 minutes.
2. Stir in all the remaining ingredients except the butter.

3. Cover and secure the lid. Turn its pressure release handle to the sealing position.
4. Cook on the "Manual" function with high pressure for 7 minutes.
5. After the beep, do a Natural release for 7 minutes.
6. Stir in butter and let it melt into the rice.
7. Serve warm.

Nutrition Values Per Serving:

Calories: 423

Carbohydrate: 66g

Protein: 7.8g

Fat: 14.9g

Sugar: 5.9g

Sodium: 298mg

Yellow Potato Rice

Serving: 3

Preparation Time: 5 minutes

Cooking Time: 12 minutes

Ingredients

- 1 cup basmati rice, rinsed
- 1 ½ tablespoons olive oil
- ½ large onion, diced small
- Salt, to taste
- 3 medium-sized potatoes, diced
- 1 ½ tablespoons chopped cilantro stalks
- 1 large garlic clove, finely diced
- ½ teaspoon turmeric powder
- 1 cup chicken stock
- 1 teaspoon butter

Directions

1. Add the oil and all the vegetables to the Instant Pot and "Sauté" for 5 minutes.
2. Stir in all the remaining ingredients except the butter.
3. Cover and secure the lid. Turn its pressure release handle to the sealing position.
4. Cook on the "Manual" function with high pressure for 7 minutes.

5. After the beep, do a Natural release for 7 minutes.
6. Stir in butter and let it melt into the rice.
7. Serve warm.

Nutrition Values Per Serving:

Calories: 466

Carbohydrate: 86.1g

Protein: 9g

Fat: 9.2g

Sugar: 3.9g

Sodium: 339mg

Mung Bean Curry

Serving: 4

Preparation Time: 10 minutes

Cooking Time: 25 minutes

Ingredients

- ½ cup raw mung beans
- 1 ½ tablespoons cooking oil
- ½ cup chopped onions
- 1 bay leaf
- ½ tablespoon grated garlic
- ¼ tablespoon grated ginger
- ¾ cup water
- 1 cup vegetable broth
- ¼ teaspoon turmeric
- ½ teaspoon coriander powder
- 1 teaspoon chili powder
- 1 cup chopped baby spinach
- Salt, to taste
- Boiled white rice to serve

Directions

1. Add the oil and onions to the Instant Pot. “Sauté” for 5 minutes.

2. Stir in ginger, garlic paste and bay leaf. Cook for 1 minute, then add all the spices.
3. Add the mung beans, broth and water to the pot.
4. Cover and secure the lid. Turn its pressure release handle to the sealing position.
5. Cook on the "Manual" function with high pressure for 15 minutes.
6. After the beep, do a Natural release for 20 minutes.
7. Stir in spinach and cook for 3 minutes on the "Sauté" setting.
8. Serve hot with boiled white rice.

Nutrition Values Per Serving:

Calories: 158

Carbohydrate: 19.2g

Protein: 8g

Fat: 5.9g

Sugar: 2.6g

Sodium: 248mg

Chickpea Tacos

Serving: 6

Preparation Time: 10 minutes

Cooking Time: 31 minutes

Ingredients

- ½ cup raw chickpeas
- 1 ½ tablespoons cooking oil
- ½ cup chopped onions
- ½ tablespoon grated garlic
- ¼ tablespoon grated ginger
- ¾ cup water
- ½ cup fresh tomato puree
- ½ green chili, finely chopped
- ¼ teaspoon turmeric
- ½ teaspoon coriander powder
- 1 teaspoon chili powder
- ½ carrot, shredded
- ½ cup green bell pepper, sliced
- Salt, to taste
- 1 tablespoon fresh cilantro to garnish (optional
- 6 tortillas

Directions

1. Add the oil and onions to the Instant Pot. "Sauté" for 5 minutes.
2. Stir in ginger, garlic paste and green chili. Cook for 1 minute, then add all the spices.
3. Add the chickpeas, tomato puree and water to the pot.
4. Cover and secure the lid. Turn its pressure release handle to the sealing position.
5. Cook on the "Manual" function with high pressure for 15 minutes.
6. After the beep, do a Natural release for 20 minutes.
7. Stir in shredded carrots and bell pepper. Cook for 10 minutes on the "Sauté" setting.
8. Fill the tortillas with prepared filling and serve.

Nutrition Values Per Serving:

Calories: 165

Carbohydrate: 25.7g

Protein: 5.3g

Fat: 5.3g

Sugar: 4.3g

Sodium: 58mg

Three-Bean Stew

Serving: 3

Preparation Time: 10 minutes

Cooking Time: 20 minutes

Ingredients

- ½ tablespoon olive oil
- ½ medium white onion, diced
- ½ medium carrot, diced into small cubes
- ½ celery stick, diced into cubes
- 3 garlic cloves, diced finely
- 1 bay leaf
- ½ teaspoon paprika powder
- ¾ teaspoon cumin powder
- ¼ teaspoon salt
- ⅛ teaspoon cinnamon powder
- ⅛ teaspoon chili powder or cayenne pepper
- ¼ cup black beans, soaked and rinsed
- ¼ cup red beans, soaked and rinsed
- ¼ cup white beans, soaked and rinsed
- ¼ cup chopped tinned tomatoes
- 2 tablespoons lemon juice
- 2 cups vegetable stock

Directions

1. Add the oil, onion, celery and garlic to the Instant Pot and "Sauté" for 5 minutes.
2. Add all the remaining ingredients to the cooker.
3. Cover and secure the lid. Turn its pressure release handle to the sealing position.
4. Cook on the "Manual" function with high pressure for 15 minutes.
5. After the beep, do a Natural release and remove the lid.
6. Stir and serve.

Nutrition Values Per Serving:

Calories: 213

Carbohydrate: 35.6g

Protein: 12g

Fat: 3.3g

Sugar: 3.6g

Sodium: 251mg

Corn Lentil Stew

Serving: 3

Preparation Time: 10 minutes

Cooking Time: 20 minutes

Ingredients

- ½ medium onion, chopped
- ½ tablespoon olive oil
- 1 medium carrot, sliced
- 3 ½ cups water
- ⅓ cup dried lentils
- 1 medium tomato
- ½ cup fresh or frozen corn
- 1 tablespoon tamari or soy sauce
- ½ cup cooked brown rice
- Salt and pepper, to taste

Directions

1. Add the oil, onion and carrots to the Instant Pot and "Sauté" for 5 minutes.
2. Add the water, lentils, tomatoes and corn to the cooker.
3. Cover and secure the lid. Turn its pressure release handle to the sealing position.
4. Cook on the "Manual" function with high pressure for 15 minutes.

5. After the beep, do a Natural release and remove the lid.
6. Stir in cooked rice, tamari sauce, salt and pepper.
7. Serve warm.

Nutrition Values Per Serving:

Calories: 239

Carbohydrate: 47.4g

Protein: 10.1g

Fat: 1.5g

Sugar: 4.2g

Sodium: 367mg

CPSIA information can be obtained
at www.ICGtesting.com
Printed in the USA
LVHW020756270422
717291LV00014B/486

9 781804 506042